The Community Health Worker

The Community Health Worker

Effective Programmes for Developing Countries

edited by

STEPHEN FRANKEL

with the assistance of
Marie-Anne Doggett

Oxford · New York · Tokyo
OXFORD UNIVERSITY PRESS
1992

Oxford University Press, Walton Street, Oxford OX2 6DP
Oxford New York Toronto
Delhi Bombay Calcutta Madras Karachi
Petaling Jaya Singapore Hong Kong Tokyo
Nairobi Dar es Salaam Cape Town
Melbourne Auckland
and associated companies in
Berlin Ibadan

Oxford is a trade mark of Oxford University Press

Published in the United States
by Oxford University Press, New York

A catalogue record for this book
is available from the British Library

Library of Congress Cataloging in Publication Data
The Community health worker : effective programmes for developing countries / edited by Stephen Frankel ; with the assistance of Marie-Anne Doggett.
Includes bibliographical references and index.
1. Community health aides. I. Frankel, Stephen. II. Doggett, Marie-Anne.
[DNLM: 1. Community Health Aides. 2. Community Health Services. 3. Developing Countries. 4. Health Policy. 5. Program Evaluation. WA 546.1 C734]
RA771.C66 1992 362.1'2'091724—dc20 91-32170
ISBN 0-19-262236-6 (hbk)
0-19-261761-3 (pbk)

Typeset by Cambridge Composing (UK) Ltd
Printed in India
by Rekha Printers Pvt. Ltd., New Delhi 110 020

Acknowledgement

This work was initiated in collaboration with Dr E. Tarimo, Director of the Division for Strengthening Health Services, World Health Organization. We should like to thank Dr Tarimo for his support and insightful comment during the preparation of this volume.

Contents

Contributors

Peter Berman, Department of Population and International Health, Harvard School of Public Health, 665 Huntingdon Avenue, Boston, Massachusetts 02115, USA.

Edward Coyle, South Glamorgan Health Authority, Temple of Peace and Health, Cathays Park, Cardiff CF1 3NW.

George Davey Smith, London School of Hygiene and Tropical Medicine, Keppel Street, London WC1E 7HT.

P. B. Desai, Gujarat Vidyapith, Ahmadabad 380014, India.

Stephen Frankel, Department of Epidemiology and Public Health Medicine, University of Bristol, Canynge Hall, Whiteladies Road, Bristol BS8 2PR.

Kris Heggenhougen, Department of Social Medicine, Harvard Medical School, 25 Shattuck Street, Boston, Massachusetts 02115, USA.

Xuegui Kan, Department of Health Inspection, Ministry of Public Health, 44 Houhai Beiyan Beijing, People's Republic of China.

Carl Kendall, Center for International Community-based Health Research, School of Hygiene and Public Health, The Johns Hopkins University, 615 North Wolfe Street, Baltimore, Maryland 21205, USA.

Claudia McConnell, Department of International Community Health, Liverpool School of Tropical Medicine, Pembroke Place, Liverpool L3 5QA.

F. M. Magari, UNFPA, Matsalamat Mansion, PO Box 9182, Dar es Salaam, Tanzania.

David Sanders, Department of Community Medicine, Faculty of Medicine, University of Zimbabwe, PO Box A178, Avondele, Harare, Zimbabwe.

Peter Sandiford, Department of International Community Health, Liverpool School of Tropical Medicine, Pembroke Place, Liverpool L3 5QA.

Mary Taylor, The International Centre for the Prevention and Treatment of Major Childhood Diseases, P. O. Box 168, Hanover, New Hampshire 03755, USA.

Acronyms

AFYA	Tanzanian Ministry of Health
AID	Agency for International Development
AMPRONAC	Nicaraguan Women's Organization
ANM	Auxiliary Nurse Midwife
APHA	American Public Health Association
APO	Aid Post Orderly
AWARE	Action for Welfare and Awakening in Rural Environment (India)
BCG	*Bacillus Calmette–Guérin* vaccine
BKKBN	National Family Planning Coordinating Board (Indonesia)
BNMT	Britain Nepal Medical Trust
CCM	Chama Cha Mapinduzi (Tanzania)
CDS	Sandinista Defence/Neighbourhood Committees (Nicaragua)
CEDHA	Centre for Educational Development in Health—Arusha (Tanzania)
CELADE	Centro Latinoamericano de Demografía (Nicaragua)
CESAMO	Centro de Salud Medico (Honduras)
CESAR	Centro de Salud Auxiliar (Honduras)
CHC	Christian Medical College and Hospital (India)
CHL	Community Health Leader
CHV	Community Health Volunteer
CHW	Community Health Worker
CNJPS	Coordinacion Nacional de las Jornadas Populares de Salud (Nicaragua)
CP	Constructive Programme (India)
CSFP	Children's Supplementary Feeding Programme (Zimbabwe)
CSU	Central Service Unit
DDCP	Diarrhoeal Disease Control Programme (Zimbabwe)

DECOPS	Division of Education and Popular Communication (Nicaragua)
DMA	Department of Medical Administration
DMO	District Medical Officer
DPHO	District Public Health Office
DPT	Diphtheria/Pertussis/Tetanus vaccine
EDENH	Encuesta Demografico Nacional de Honduras
EPC	Evaluation and Planning Centre (London School of Hygiene and Tropical Medicine)
FCV	Family Care Volunteer
FESOMENIC	Nicaraguan Doctors' Medical Association
FETSALUD	Nicaraguan Health Workers' Trade Union
FPAI	Family Planning Association of India
FSLN	Frente Sandinista de Liberacion Nacional (Nicaragua)
GCEP	Goitre and Cretinism Eradication Project (Nepal)
HA	Health Aide (China and India)/Health Assistant (Zimbabwe)
HG	Health Guardian (Honduras)/Health Guide (India)
HMG	His Majesty's Government (Nepal)
HR	Health Representative
ICHSDP	Integrated Community Health Services Development Project (Nepal)
ICMR	Indian Council of Medical Research
ICSSR	Indian Council of Social Science Research
IMR	Infant Mortality Rate
INAA	Ministry of Water Supply and Drainage (Nicaragua)
INEC	Instituto Nacional de Estadisticas y Cenos (Nicaragua)
IU(C)D	Intra-Uterine (Contraceptive) Device
KHARDEP	Kosi Hill Area Rural Development Programme (Nepal)
MA	Medical Assistant
MCCD	Ministry of Community and Cooperative Development (Zimbabwe)
MCCDWA	Ministry of Community and Cooperative Development and Women's Affairs (Zimbabwe)
MCH	Maternal and Child Health
MIDINDRA	Ministry of Agriculture and Agrarian Reform (Nicaragua)

MINSA	Ministerio de Salud (Nicaragua)
MINVAH	Ministerio de Viviendas y Asentamientos Humanos (Nicaragua)
MOH	Ministry of Health
MOPH	Ministry of Public Health
MPW	Multi-Purpose Worker
NGO	Non Governmental Organization
NPC	National Planning Committee (India)
NWO	Nepal Women's Organization
ORS/T	Oral Rehydration Salts/Therapy
PBCCPCC	Political Bureau of the Chinese Communist Party Central Committee
PHC	Primary Health Care
PIAAS	Programa Integral de Atencion en las Areas de Salud (Nicaragua)
PMOH	Provincial Medical Officer of Health
PNS	Plan Nacional de Salud (Honduras)
PSU	Peripheral Service Unit
RCO	Rural Community Organizer
RUHSA	Rural Unit for Health and Social Affairs (India)
SIDA	Swedish International Development Authority
TANU	Tanganyika African National Union
TCDV	Technical Cooperation among Developing Villages
TM	Traditional Midwife
TTLs	Tribal Trust Lands
UN	United Nations
UNESCO	United Nations Educational, Scientific and Cultural Organization
UNICEF	United Nations International Children's Emergency Fund
UPASI	United Planters Association of Southern India
UPGK	Programme to Improve Family Nutrition (Indonesia)
USAID	United States Agency for International Development
VCW	Village Community Worker
VHC	Village Health Committee
VHP	Village Health Post
VHW	Village Health Worker

VIDCO	Village Development Committee
WADCO	Ward Development Committee
WHC	Ward Health Committee
WHO	World Health Organization
ZANU (PF)	Zimbabwe African National Union (Patriotic Front)
ZEPI	Zimbabwe Expanded Programme on Immunization
ZNFPC	Zimbabwe National Family Planning Council

1
Overview
STEPHEN FRANKEL

Community health workers (CHWs) have achieved much in many countries at different times, but the frequent disappointment with the outcome of CHW programmes is often attributed to inadequacies in the CHW concept, or even laid at the door of the CHWs themselves. This debate is a sterile one. There is no longer any place for discussion of *whether* CHWs can be key actors in achieving adequate health care. The question is *how* to achieve their potential.

With this in mind, the contributors to this book have sought to provide an overview of the situation in their countries, by documenting experiences and offering informed observations on the way forward as they see it. The chapters represent a wide-ranging analysis of the achievements and difficulties of CHWs in Africa, South America, Asia, and Indonesia, and it is hoped that such a broad approach will contribute significantly to an understanding of the present position and an appreciation of future requirements.

This introductory chapter seeks to synthesize some of the conclusions to be drawn from the vast literature which has accumulated on the implementation of CHW programmes throughout the world. The CHW provides an ideal bridge between the community and the health sector. However, experience in numerous countries has demonstrated that top priority must be given to understanding and tackling the problems raised by attempting to achieve this bridging function in practice. CHWs are variously regarded as extenders of health services and agents for educational and developmental change (Walt 1990). If they are to be more than an 'extra pair of hands' or an 'additional element', however welcome, then countries must show themselves more committed to structural change than has hitherto been apparent (Ramprasad 1988).

This view is re-echoed by McConnell and Taylor (pp. 102–24)

whose exposé of the introduction of the Community Health Volunteer (CHV) programme in Nepal cites an example where mistakes have been made but no lessons have been learnt because major structural and administrative constraints remain in conflict with implementation pressures for decentralization. From India's experience, Desai (pp. 125–55) also concludes that the main need is to resurrect socially and economically shattered community organizations so that they can make better use of the available CHWs.

The widespread difficulty in achieving the undoubted potential of this category of worker stems not from medical or other technical problems, but from organizational and management issues, which are analysed here both in relation to the community and in relation to other priorities for strengthening district primary health care (PHC). The considerable experience which has now built up around the more circumscribed choices involved in mobilizing CHWs are also collated, such as those concerning their job descriptions, methods of payment, coverage, working hours, recruitment, training, and career structure. Finally, the issues raised by the need for effective monitoring and evaluation of CHW programmes are addressed since it is not possible to learn constructively from them unless this function is adequately performed.

THE PAST AND FUTURE OF COMMUNITY HEALTH WORKERS

The term 'community health worker' only came into use in the 1980s, and in many parts of the world they are still known by other names, such as 'family welfare educators', 'health promoters', 'health volunteers' (Walt 1990), 'community health aides' (Haraldson 1988), or 'village health workers' (VHWs) (Capps and Crane 1989; Matomora 1989).

The definition of CHWs adopted by the 1986 Yaoundé Conference was that they should be 'members of the communities where they work; should be selected by the communities; should be answerable to the communities for their activities; should be supported by the health system but not necessarily a part of its organization; and have a shorter training than professional workers' (WHO 1987). The momentum in the mobilization of CHWs is increasing world-wide as it becomes more generally accepted that the wide deployment of generalist health workers is the main avenue towards achieving PHC in most countries.

CHW programmes are seen as encompassing all of the Alma-Ata principles (WHO 1978*a*), but there is a danger that in some countries they may be *equated* with PHC (WHO Study Group 1989) rather than comprising a part of it (Walt 1988). The introduction of CHWs into India has not been accompanied by any departure from the proliferation of health infrastructures, nor by any change in attitudes and vested interests—a situation which has led Desai (pp. 125–55) to propose what he describes as an 'alternative approach to Health for All in rural India'.

When success in PHC is expressed in terms of the numbers of CHWs trained, rather than in the quality of their performance (Mburu and Boerma 1989), then 'health for all' becomes 'CHWs for all' and the primary health care strategy is 'robbed of its spirit and power' (Matomora 1989).

There is, of course, nothing new about using health workers whose training and education are less than that considered adequate for full professional status (Fendall 1972; Fendall and Tiwari 1980). This has long been common practice in military medicine, as well as in colonial health services. However, the emphasis upon using such workers is now somewhat different. Earlier use was justified mainly on the grounds of expediency. Health workers with a higher educational level were seen as desirable, but, in the absence of such trainees or the resources to pay them, it was acceptable to train candidates with limited educational experience. Now the emphasis is upon the positive value and unique benefits of such recruits. Their lack of professional qualification is seen as a positive asset, as one expression of the lack of distance between these workers and the people they serve. In Tanzania, Heggenhougen and Magari (pp. 156–77) recall that CHWs were originally seen as a stop-gap, but are now recognized as a permanent feature, while in Zimbabwe, Sanders (pp. 178–219) reminds us that one of the main problems of the government VHW programmes was that of unwanted over-professionalization.

Interest in and advocacy of CHWs thus has two sets of origins. The first stems from the past failure of health-centre-based services to provide adequate coverage of services appropriate to the major health problems at practicable cost. The second is the acknowledgement that simple technical measures to combat disease can have only a partial impact upon conditions that are explicable largely in terms of environmental, social, and cultural issues. Tackling health problems in isolation from such factors is now considered 'a thing of the past' (Backett 1989), and CHWs offer one potential point of entry for influencing these precursors of illness, providing they are 'immersed in their cultural context' (Bastien 1990). From Honduras, Kendall (pp. 241–60) reports that the main reason for the failure of implementation of the programmes he describes stems from an ignorance of, and lack of respect for, the socio-cultural context of rural attitudes and perceptions.

The East African experience (Mburu and Boerma 1989) illustrates some of the socio-economic and political problems which have to be taken into account. Both Kan (pp. 88–101) in China and Sanders in Zimbabwe (pp. 178–219) emphasize the centrality of politics and socio-economic organization to health and health care organization. However, various barriers to effective health services may be overcome through the mobilization of CHWs, who can reduce the geographical, social, and cultural distance between the services and their target population, concentrate upon the sorts of changes that influence the true nature of the health problem, and achieve these aims within acceptable costs.

These separate strands in the origins of current advocacy of CHWs correspond with two distinct elements in their potential contribution. On the one hand, these workers are in a position to offer basic health services to populations otherwise denied access to medical treatments for life-threatening or discomforting illnesses. This role corresponds with their origin as a response to the massive unmet demand for conventional health services in many countries. On the other hand, they are the potential agents of the sort of community participation in health that is essential for tackling the wider precursors of illness.

While these two sets of functions for CHWs are usually combined in the one person, it is helpful to keep these components of their contribution analytically distinct. Conceptually, one can view CHWs' contributions as stretching along a continuum, with the provision of simple treatments at one pole and the promotion of health at the other. Such promotive activities may range from advocating simple preventive measures to fostering wider community development. Activities at the curative pole represent the furthest outreach of conventional health services, while those at the promotive pole are expressions of the broader concept of health care that was expressed in the Alma-Ata Declaration (WHO 1978*a*). The particular position of each country's CHWs along this continuum will vary according to the level of development and the penetration of conventional health services. The curative role may be less relevant where such demands are readily met by the formal health sector. The promotive role is potentially relevant to countries at all levels of development.

This then is the potential place of the CHW. It is a formidable job description. Is there any evidence that CHWs are effective in these roles? A number of evaluations of special projects are available (for example, Alderman *et al.* 1973; Berggren *et al.* 1981; Kielmann *et al.* 1978; Haliman and Williams 1983; Capps and Crane 1989; Bastien 1990), from which there appears to be no doubt that the activities of CHWs can effect major changes in mortality and other indices of health status. They can also satisfy prominent felt needs that cannot realistically be met by other means. There is therefore no need to discuss whether CHW programmes *can* be effective.

When the focus moves to national programmes, however, the picture becomes rather different. The available evidence concerning CHW activities is largely unsatisfactory for formal evaluation, since the bulk of this literature is concerned with advocacy rather than analysis, and, in the main, talks about CHWs rather than to them or their clients. However, what does emerge is the inescapable conclusion that in almost all areas CHWs are failing to achieve the contribution which is clearly their potential, and which is an essential pre-condition of health for all. This point is reiterated by Berman (pp. 62–87) in describing the Indonesian programme, and by other contributors to this book.

Reproducing successful small projects on a national scale remains a serious problem, as illustrated by both Desai in India, when describing the AWARE and RUHSA projects (pp. 142–6), and Sanders in his account of the Bondolfi Mission programme in Zimbabwe (pp. 197–9), and over-optimism about the role of CHWs, is tending to undermine their potential (Walt 1990). In Ecuador, for example, operational problems have hampered the smooth functioning of the programme, despite initial optimism (Mangelsdorf 1988).

A recent report from a WHO Study Group (1989) identified eight areas of weakness, the overwhelming majority of which stem from the social, cultural, and management issues that are the necessary and inevitable consequence of the CHWs' structural position at the interface between the health sector and the local population. Failure to acknowledge these issues fully can only result in an ineffective programme and wasted resources. An analysis of the various aspects of the CHWs' structural position is therefore imperative.

CHWS IN THE CONTEXT OF DISTRICT PHC

The design and execution of effective CHW programmes raise a number of technical issues concerning specific means of tackling identified health problems, but the resolution of such questions is a relatively minor problem compared to the organizational issues which are raised by CHW programmes at the district level. The critical obstacles to effective CHW programmes are to be found in this area, and it is here that even the most committed programmes may founder. Such questions are necessary consequences of the structural position of CHWs. In social terms, these workers occupy the space at the interface between the health sector and the local population. In cultural terms, they straddle differences between indigenous and cosmopolitan views of illness, as illustrated by Kendall in Honduras (pp. 241–60), and tensions within cosmopolitan medicine between cure and prevention, as illustrated by Heggenhougen and Magari in Tanzania (pp. 156–77).

National perspectives

Before considering the influences of the local social milieu upon the functioning of CHWs, it is important to stress the prior importance of the wider stage. A key issue here is political will. CHW programmes are most likely to succeed where they are an expression of a conscious political choice to promote the living standards of the less advantaged sections of the population (Bossert and Parker 1984). Improvements in health status relate to the wider social, cultural, and physical environment. A national commitment to an equitable distribution of resources may facilitate a variety of improvements including the deployment of well-supported CHWs, but appropriate political support is by no means the only factor. The experience in Nicaragua (pp. 220–40) is an instructive example of the possibilities and limitations of a PHC strategy, even when political will was present at the highest governmental level.

Nevertheless, it is possible for CHWs to be effective even in less fortuitous circumstances (Haliman and Williams 1983; Islam and Bachman 1983), in which the promotion of CHWs can constitute a political statement. When the intention of promoting CHWs is to influence the broader precursors of ill health, their activities are likely to highlight those aspects of environmental disadvantage that relate to inequality (Stark 1985). This sort of activity can expose the effective CHW to personal danger (Chowdhury 1981; Werner and Bower 1982), perhaps nowhere more so than in war-torn El Salvador (Capps and Crane 1989), and of course, in Nicaragua (pp. 220–40).

A more circumscribed political issue concerns the potential threat that CHWs may represent to other groups of health workers. Relationships between CHWs, doctors, and especially nurses, are acknowledged as a key feature for success in Bolivia (Bastien 1990), and firm team-work is of the essence in Alaska (Haraldson 1988). Conversely in India, integration of the CHWs is considered to be hampered by the bias of other health professionals (Ramprasad 1988), whom Desai (pp. 125–55) describes as over-bureaucratic and 'too professional'. Both doctors and nurses can oppose the dispensing of basic drugs by CHWs and there may be role strains, particularly when nurses are not involved in planning programmes and do not understand the cultural beliefs of the workers they may nevertheless be expected to train (Walt 1990). In Nicaragua, Coyle, Davey Smith, and Sandiford (pp. 220–40) report that attempts to introduce more specialized roles for the voluntary CHWs in 1984 were foiled by the control exercised by salaried professionals, especially Auxiliary Nurses.

The community

Planning documents have about them a neatness and symmetry which is quite lacking on the ground. The basic structures may accord with planned intentions, but as the service spreads further from the centre it is likely to take on the complexion of the local scene. This structural separation of the periphery from the centre is a necessary feature of a widely accessible health service, but many of the problems that beset health programmes follow from this truism.

In addition to those aspects of the social environment which influence the practical running of a service, the sorts of decisions individuals make in relation to activities that may influence health and illness are also guided by a variety of local characteristics. People do not make uniform or predictable use of the variety of resources for prevention, cure, or care that may be available to them, as illustrated by Kendall's case-study in Honduras (pp. 241–60). A variety of factors, including cost, personal preference based upon past experience of efficacy, the expectation of a sympathetic hearing, the recommendation of others, and so on, influence these choices.

The CHW is adrift in these choppy seas, and without some sort of anchoring within the formal system it is unlikely that his or her efforts will be directed effectively towards the measures which may be expected to produce significant benefit to health status.

While the variety of detailed circumstances is as varied as the range of societies, cultures, and environments where CHWs are active, there is striking similarity between common types of problems that emerge. Some important generalizations are therefore possible. First, these concern issues that centre upon aspects of the social relationships which may influence the effectiveness of CHWs, and second, aspects of the wider local medical scene within which CHW activities must be viewed.

Community involvement

The sort of community alluded to in much of the literature about 'community participation' is at best an idealization and at worst a misleading myth. The word community can mean simply a number of people living in the same area, but it also carries the implications of common interests and fellowship. McConnell and Taylor (pp. 102–24) cite Nepal as a good example of a country in which there is such great geographical and political diversity that few village 'communities' can be identified, either physically or culturally.

In fact, a community is not a 'homogeneous entity' in which all the members live in the same way, with the same interests and aspirations, but rather an entity in which the importance of social class dynamics must be acknowledged (Tumwine 1989). In practice, social groupings at this level co-operate selectively and in particular contexts. The political process which leads to particular projects gaining support and others wilting through inaction, is a complex and often unpredictable one. In a national programme the potential for the preferred outcome in each locality is therefore uncertain.

Case studies illustrate the complexities of these processes in differing social environments. An account of an Indonesian programme illustrates the problems that may follow from the political implications of introducing new health workers (Williams and Satoto 1983). An account from Papua New Guinea illustrates the problems that can arise when the 'community' served by a CHW consists of a number of social groupings that have no tradition of maintained co-operation. There the aid post may serve a number of parishes while necessarily being sited in only one of them. Traditionally, there may have been temporary or even long-term alliances between the parishes in relation to major political concerns. But in everyday affairs the parish itself does not function as a corporate body, and there would be no routine co-operation between parishes. In practice, the action group is ordered around each individual's personal network of relations and friends, and conflicts between such groupings may find expression in disputes about access to health services (Frankel 1984).

Where the resources for a particular activity are also scarce, or have to be raised largely by local effort, the likelihood of success becomes smaller still. In Nepal, where there are no clear plans for switching to community funding and no real village-level orientation, there are fears that motivation will be lost (McConnell and Taylor, pp. 102–24). In Zambia, an intensive local study detailed tensions caused by the failure of some of the villages to provide remuneration for the CHW (Twumasi and Freund 1985).

The ambiguous position of CHWs between the community and the health sector may lead to conflicts of interest in attempting to please either party. For example, in the CHW scheme in India it was found that health centre staff valued CHWs' support in areas such as family planning, where villagers were reluctant to come forward (Maru 1983). Such involvement in an unpopular programme must have caused a strong identification of the CHW with government rather than community aspirations. Desai (pp. 125–55) considers that the whole Rural Health Scheme has been undermined by this association with family-planning propaganda.

CHWs are, by definition, marginal to both the formal health care system on the one hand, and the social setting of health care on the other. This marginal role between the community and the health sector can lead to their acceptance by neither. The 'conflicting views as to whether a CHW should represent the community or the health sector' reported from India (WHO 1986*a*) express the difficulty of achieving the ideal, which would be to represent both. From this, given that they straddle the borderline between these two universes of health care, follow both their strengths and their weaknesses. The very title, community health worker, could be seen as a terminological attempt to gloss over the tension inherent in this marginal position. Progress can only be achieved by acknowledging this tension, in order to attempt harnessing it where possible or defusing it where not.

These case studies illustrate the misleading nature of the naïve view of the word 'community'. It must therefore be assumed that a CHW is serving not a solitary social grouping of unified purpose, but a population whose commitment to particular projects will vary according to their perceptions of benefit and the social and political context of the activity. From here on, the word community is therefore used in the geographical sense of the population potentially served by a CHW. There is no assumption that such social groupings co-operate harmoniously in everyday affairs.

Genuine community participation cannot be built into a programme in any predictable way. This is the paradox of centrally prompted community participation, and may be a particular danger when programmes are sponsored by non-governmental donors, whose own participation is then often substituted for that of the community (Tarimo and Fowkes 1989). From Zimbabwe, Sanders (pp. 178–219) devotes a large part of his chapter to an understanding of the crucial role played by the interlocking of State and popular organizations in the process of community participation.

The process of involvement necessarily raises the likelihood that communities' perceptions of need will not coincide with those of health personnel. Geunine community participation must involve respecting such divergencies, including the rejection of CHWs where communities feel that their resources should be directed to developments seen as more pressing. For example, in Indonesia, a doctor who wished to interest people in a voluntary health insurance scheme found that people were more interested in investing in an irrigation dam (Haliman and Williams 1983). When villagers in Papua New Guinea were asked their priorities, they said that they wanted a road rather than an expanded health programme. Nevertheless, in the Indonesian example, co-operation over the dam led to a broad-based development and health programme, which illustrates the longer-term benefits that may follow genuine participation.

These issues must be acknowledged as inescapable facets of any CHW programme. Nevertheless, it is also the case that community involvement is an essential component of any radical programme of health improvement. In planning terms, the key to the facilitation of constructive community involvement lies in the creation and support of a variety of links between the centre and the periphery. The nature and potential of these aspects of strengthening district PHC are analysed below.

Relationships with other healing systems

Here it is more difficult to generalize. The general aim of a working partnership between the formal health care system and traditional practices has a varying relevance according to particular national or local circumstances. Kendall (pp. 241–60) considers that modifications are necessary to Ministry of Health (MOH) policy in Honduras to take account of the centrality of folk medicine to the rural communities he describes. Such a partnership is more common where strong advocacy of the place of traditional medicine is found at the national political level, as in China (Signer and Galston 1972), and India (Leslie 1976). Elsewhere, traditional medicine is seemingly not strongly represented in CHW programmes.

The 'state of the art' study (American Public Health Association 1977) found that indigenous healers were being trained in 8 per cent of projects only. The content of this training or the planned role of the trainees was not investigated. More recently, there are signs that mediation between traditional and modern medicine is receiving more attention, at least in Bolivia, where as many as one-quarter of new trainees were selected from among traditional practitioners in a recent project (Bastien 1990).

The aim of integrating cosmopolitan and traditional medical systems is often talked of loosely as a guiding principle of CHW programmes, but it is important to scrutinize what is meant by this in practice. Western, scientific, or cosmopolitan, medicine can indeed be seen as a system. It is underpinned by a single set of assumptions and is made available to people through an identifiable organizational structure, which is visible to people and in most respects external to their own social networks. Indigenous means of interpreting and responding to illness are in general quite different. A variety of choices are available to people, including eliciting the services of specialist healers, but where other major traditions such as *Ayurvedic* medicine are not prominent, there is in general no single overarching organizational scheme. Instead, people are guided in preventive as well as curative practices by a set of concepts that explain risk, provide means of protection, and inform the treatment of particular ailments.

Different individuals may be more or less knowledgeable and some may specialize as healers, but the management of an illness is almost always determined by the decisions of those close to a patient. In so far as a 'traditional system' has any organizational coherence, this usually centres upon the activities of a 'therapy management group' (Janzen 1979), which will call upon the services of different sorts of practitioners, including modern ones, as appropriate. It is therefore rare for traditional healing to have any permanent structure which the modern sector can tap. Rather, it is more usually the case that the initiative is taken by kin who mobilise particular cures as they see fit.

Healers may or may not be suitable candidates for CHW training. Where individuals respected for their abilities in healing are able and willing to take on this additional role there are clear advantages in training them; for example, the majority of CHWs trained in a programme in Sarawak were Iban healers (Chen and Tan 1981). However, in some circumstances there may be strong reasons why they should not be considered. In Botswana, the healing power of some types of healer is thought to be complemented by their power to harm through sorcery, which renders them unwelcome colleagues for Christian nurses (Barbee 1986). In India, an earlier positive view of traditional practitioners was reversed when it was found that 'their own interests were in conflict with the objectives of the CHW scheme' (WHO 1984).

While formal integration between the health care sector and traditional practitioners may be problematic in some areas, it is important to remember that from the user's point of view such organizationally distinct sets of facilities and expertise may appear complementary. From the point of view of the consumer there is not necessarily any conflict between the traditional sector and cosmopolitan medicine. It is well known that medical pluralism, where people shuttle between the various options open to them, is the norm in most countries (Janzen 1978; Kleinman 1980; Frankel 1986; Frankel and Lewis 1989).

In considering the issue of such integration it is important to stress the crucial difference between the conceptual frameworks that underpin traditional medical systems and the body of empirical techniques offered by traditional practitioners; that is, the difference between traditional medicines and traditional medicine. The model for the integration of traditional and cosmopolitan medicine is often held to be the Chinese system. However, what happened in China was that particular traditional therapeutic practices, often modified for incorporation into modern practice, were offered by barefoot doctors as options within their therapeutic repertoire. Concepts of the disequilibrium of the elements and other fundamental tenets of the traditional system were not incorporated into barefoot doctors' activities, so that medical practice was conducted largely according to allopathic principles (Bibeau 1985). Such appropriation of a few traditional techniques or herbs, or the inclusion of a number of traditional practitioners in a CHW programme, is perhaps of less relevance to PHC than the need to integrate people's traditional means for pursuing health with the ideas of preventive medicine.

Where integration is certainly necessary is in harnessing traditional concepts to inform plans for behavioural change. There are usually clear parallels between concerns that are informed by knowledge of the natural history of disease and those of traditional medical thought. Limited success in promotive activities relates to the failure to incorporate scientific ideas into peoples' own frame of reference, as is well known. CHWs are well-placed to achieve this bridging function, although it must be remembered that they are also likely to share with their clients any misconceptions about the relevance or value of changes informed by scientific principles (Frankel and Lehmann 1984).

However, the educational implications of people's own views of health and illness are perhaps less important than the organizational implications. Health is valued, but it is a common observation that 'health services' are not supported in the same way that some other institutions are. One explanation for this is that other activities to do with subsistence, moral welfare, or education are seen as offering more in terms of broad-based benefit, while health services are in practice seen as 'illness services'. Whether household budgets are very limited or not it is common for people to give priority to these other activities until such time as illness actively threatens.

This common indifference to 'health' services in times of health is an indication of the fact that the broader interest of communities in health is situated outside the 'health' sector. Primary health care demands that this universal concern with well-being is guided towards changes that are known to be medically beneficial. Just as the sort of preventive measures that are commonly proposed rarely result in an energetic response, 'health' issues often fail to stimulate organizational support in the way that other concerns such as education, irrigation, or religious affairs may. These issues are highly relevant to the effectiveness of the CHW. For true community support to be forthcoming it may be necessary to seek co-operation in the context of the wider concerns of the people. This is an added argument for intersectoral co-operation. Not only is such co-operation an important avenue for PHC, but it may also be a precondition for energetic community involvement.

Community health workers and the strengthening of district PHC

The constructive response to this analysis of the variety of influences likely to undermine the effectiveness of CHWs is to strengthen the district health system. Increasingly the district, with a population of between 100 000 and 300 000, is being recognized as the 'implementation unit for an integrated assault on health problems' (Tarimo and Fowkes 1989). The district health system is a key concept in the development of PHC, and it is therefore important to define what is meant by this term. The Yaoundé Conference defined it in this way:

A district health system based on primary health care is a more or less self-contained segment of the national health system. It comprises first and foremost a well-defined population, living within a clearly delineated administrative and geographical area, whether urban or rural. It includes all institutions and individuals providing health care in the district, whether governmental, social security, non-governmental, private, and traditional . . . The organization of district health systems will obviously depend on the specific situation in each country and each district, including the structure and personalities involved. Nevertheless a key feature is the mechanism for managing activities within the communities and villages and creating dialogue between the people and the health sector which leads to a process of adaptation to community needs and of learning from successes and failures.

Few districts have these mechanisms at the moment in their villages, communities or other appropriate units. The purpose of current activities is to give this capability to district systems so that effective dialogue with communities can be maintained.

The district health system is the framework for the indispensable support without which the CHW cannot function effectively and, in fact, without which the CHW scheme may fail (WHO 1987).

Thus, the outcome of CHW programmes at local level is largely determined by the nature of the links between the health sector and the community, as amply illustrated by the focus of most contributors to this book. In exceptional circumstances, communities may develop long-term activities entirely through their own initiative, and maintain these through local enthusiasm. Such programmes offer ideal examples of PHC in action, but national programmes cannot depend upon fortuitous local circumstances. Where CHW programmes are to be the vehicle for PHC, the key to success must lie in the nature of the relationship between peripheral services and the health care system that supports them. The components of such relationships that offer creative opportunities for programme development include: an organizational framework that allows joint guidance of local CHW-related activities; supervision; continuing education; an information system; referral arrangements, and a supply system. Each of these is considered in turn.

Support groups

In innumerable localities CHW services fail for reasons that in each case may appear trivial and avoidable. However, it is argued here that this multiplicity of unique circumstances follows predictably from the structural position of the CHW. Problems follow, first from current relationships between the centre and periphery, and second, from relationships at the periphery. These relationships must be given some sort of institutional framework which may counteract the fissile tendencies within each CHW area, increase the accountability of the CHW to the people he or she serves, and make events at the periphery more visible to those at the centre. Previous experience in Bolivia has shown the vital necessity of community support (Bastien 1990), and in Ecuador the presence of a health committee was a 'strong predictor of performance' (Mangelsdorf 1988).

An essential prerequisite for a viable CHW programme is therefore some sort of support group within the community served, which articulates actively with the health sector (WHO 1984). This is a fundamental requirement if the range of specific issues discussed below, such as recruitment, remuneration, the scope of the programme, and accountability, are to be resolved to mutual advantage. Such support groups are necessarily the nodal point of a CHW programme, and there is great concern in Nepal (pp. 102–24), where supervision and support strategies have been postponed in a situation which places all the emphasis on providing training. Inadequate supervision and support is 'an area of acknowledged weakness in all national programmes' and represents the greatest challenge facing them, confronted as they are by 'enormous constraints of management, where . . . rules and regulations introduced to ensure uniformity and equity . . . actually result in rigidity, immobility and demoralization' (Walt 1990).

Where viable community organizations exist, the additional functions relating to CHWs may be added to their remit. Where they do not, the task of promoting a support group underpinned both by the community and by government personnel is a problematic one. There can be no alternative to developing suitable links between the health sector and the community to 'sensitize' the community to the programme before specific tasks such as the selection of CHWs are undertaken (WHO 1984). This activity must be regarded as an early stage in a long-term commitment by health centre staff in supporting the support group.

Any PHC programme must ideally receive political support from the centre if it is to achieve its wider aims. Even where the initiative is largely local such support is important if the programme is to achieve longer-term stability. The project in Indonesia (Haliman and Williams 1983) is interesting in that the impetus came from a voluntary agency and local communities. Tensions between these communities and local government officials were defused only through the constructive support of a senior official. The opposite experience was common in the Indian CHW programme, where volunteers were appointed by village leaders and had no outside support. CHWs were not in a position to introduce changes which would be resisted by dominant groups in the village (Jobert 1985).

However, external support may also stifle genuine popular participation in health care, as when a government CHW programme in Zimbabwe undermined a local self-help scheme, and in the process rendered CHWs less accountable to those most in need of their services (Sanders 1985).

Countries differ in the extent to which support groups concern themselves solely with health issues or are responsible for a range of community development activities (WHO 1984). One issue identified in the interregional study is the need for training of support group members. The effectiveness of CHW programmes must depend to a large extent on the strength of these support groups. It is clearly essential that their members should have a realistic understanding of the place of differing strategies for health improvement, as well as possess the administrative and accounting skills required for the management of their local CHW. Such training and other tasks involved in the support of support groups are an important component of the supervision of CHWs (WHO 1987).

Supervision

The extent to which this topic is referred to as a key area of failure indicates that there are fundamental and common features to this aspect of CHW programmes. All eleven countries involved in the WHO interregional study reported that lack of interest in supervision by supervisors was a problem, and the Tanzanian experience suggests that inadequate and varied supervision still bedevils many programmes (pp. 156–77) (WHO 1984). Throughout the literature there are comments on the fact that few supervisors take their tasks seriously. Contradictions and inconsistencies can confuse CHWs, many of whom are not even sure who their supervisors actually are (WHO Study Group 1989).

This issue is particularly critical because the quantified impact of a number of pilot CHW projects must at least in part be explicable by the degree of supervision and support offered by highly motivated team leaders. For instance, in the Narangwal nutrition project, where considerable benefits were recorded, CHWs were supported by weekly visits from a doctor and a public health nurse (Kielmann *et al.* 1978). Similar considerations apply in other projects, including Jamaica (Alderman *et al.* 1973), Haiti (Berggren *et al.* 1981), and Alaska (Haraldson 1988).

Supervisors are often health centre personnel. Regular visits to health centres can allow continuing education, discussion of problems, and exchange of information, but such opportunities are often missed (WHO Study Group 1989), and supervision can all too often be equated with involving the CHW in performing routine health centre tasks (Walt 1990). It has been the experience in many countries that staff with clinical duties in health centres are likely to give a low priority to the support of CHWs. One factor here is that clinical demands tend to take precedence. It is well known that working patterns are influenced primarily by the immediate working environment. A distant and scattered body of CHWs do not make immediate demands upon a health centre worker in the same way that a queue of mothers and crying children do. Supervisory visits are often cancelled from lack of transport or motivation, and then when they do occur may be an empty ritual which can undermine the CHW more than motivate him or her. A productive balance between encouragement and assessment is less likely to be struck by supervisors who are themselves ambivalent about the task. Clinical workers are also likely to stress clinical activities, as has been reported from Botswana (WHO 1986a).

Other barriers to satisfactory supervision include the social distance between health centre staff and the communities they serve, and the reluctance to view villagers' autonomy positively, as was noted in the WHO interregional study (WHO 1984). Such attitudes are not consistent with the reorientation of the health system that is basic to PHC, so that efforts to modify them through training are to be encouraged.

These considerations indicate that assigning CHW supervision to staff with primarily clinical duties results in the supervisory role taking second place. There are therefore strong arguments for mobilizing a special cadre of CHW supervisors with sufficient training and management ability to maintain motivation in a task which has proved widely problematic. The costs of such a cadre of health workers, including their wages, transport costs, training, and other support, would fall to the health sector. This may be seen as a basic investment in any serious CHW programme. However, the manpower and financial implications are considerable, and therefore require careful planning in each case.

The issue of employing experienced CHWs in this role is discussed in the context of a career structure for CHWs. It must be stressed that this strategy of promoting the most effective CHWs to supervisory roles does not lead to a satisfactory solution where these workers are not adequately supported. It is common to find CHWs who were previously effective in their communities slipping into hollow bureaucratic roles.

However committed supervisors may be to the task, their visits can only occupy a trivial proportion of the CHW's working hours. In contrast, the CHW's clients are present all the time. Supervision in an Indonesian programme (Haliman and Williams 1983) is relevant here. It is ordered around a system of ongoing motivation where clusters of villages share in the process of setting goals and monitoring progress.

There are clear advantages to such an arrangement, though it may not be welcomed by CHWs. Their uncertainty in relation to such dual accountability is demonstrated in an investigation of the attitudes of various participants in church health programmes in Indonesia, the Philippines, and Hong Kong (Rifkin 1983). It emerged that development workers and medical professionals favoured greater responsibility for health care on the part of communities. CHWs, on the other hand, preferred the professionals to make the decisions. This in part is likely to reflect the uncertain position of these workers, and their wish for their role to be clearly supported by the expertise and authority of health professionals. Accountability to those who observe their daily activities may also be unwelcome.

Nevertheless, some sort of joint responsibility must be the ideal, where supervision is shared between the community being served and the health sector. Community supervision would concentrate upon accountability, while the health sector focuses upon more technical aspects. The success of such an arrangement will depend upon the strength and coherence of the support group, as well as its proper support by the CHW supervisor and other members of the health team. In China, Kan (pp. 88–101) reports little conflict between technical supervision and village accountability among the barefoot doctors, who were given strong political support. However, in Zimbabwe, Sanders (pp. 178–219) relates that the relationship of VHWs to the community has been marred by struggles over political accountability to the community or technical accountability to the Ministry of Health.

Continuing education

The third potential influence upon the effectiveness of CHWs is the process of continuing education. This has been an important feature of successful CHW programmes. For example, in China a structured cycle of continuing education included visits to the commune hospital, formal additional training courses on a regular basis, as well as visits to the barefoot doctor's health post from a variety of health workers, including the supervisor (Flahault 1978).

That continuing education is an essential prerequisite for an effective CHW programme is self-evident. This point requires no further discussion. However, to be successful, specific provision for this basic activity must be made. Where continuing education is regarded as ancillary to supervisory contacts, or assumed to occur on an informal basis during health centre visits, it is unlikely that CHWs are in reality receiving meaningful further training. The limited comments on continuing education in the WHO interregional study (WHO 1984) suggest that this essential component of effective CHW programmes may not be receiving sufficient attention. Statements such as 'irregularly carried out through supervision', 'periodically', 'usually 1 week per year', 'supposed to be 1 day per month, but has not succeeded', suggest that this activity has not been given the priority it requires.

As with supervision, the support of continuing education has significant resource implications for the health sector. This essential pre-condition for an effective CHW programme must therefore be given urgent consideration where it has not already been accorded the highest priority.

The information system

There is no doubt that CHWs are capable of gathering useful information, even those who have the most limited formal education. Where literacy is inadequate, tally systems have been devised (Radford 1978). However, the undoubted potential of CHWs in a variety of health-related surveillance activities must be considered in relation to the actual use that may be made of specific categories of information.

A reporting system has three main functions. The first is to provide a continuing record of care for each patient to avoid what Morley calls treatment on a 'cafeteria' basis (1973). Where such health books are held by individuals, particularly mothers, it would be proper for literate CHWs to enter a note on their assessments or treatments. This activity is unexceptional and makes only a limited demand on CHWs.

The second function of a reporting system is to supply those in charge with information on disease patterns and on the performance of health services. This is a designated function of CHWs in most of the programmes included in the WHO interregional study (WHO 1984) and is a feasible way in which to gain valuable information, though staff are seldom aware of the epidemiological value of their record-keeping (Walt 1990). Some of the issues raised by the collection of such data by workers with limited formal education are addressed in a WHO report (WHO 1978*b*). A particularly ambitious scheme is reported from Costa Rica, where information collected by CHWs 'is aggregated by district and region to form the basis of a computerized national data system, which can immediately pinpoint areas of high malnutrition or other forms of deprivation, so that additional resources can be channelled towards them' (Harrison 1981). Inevitably, the value of this sort of activity, as with all components of CHW programmes, depends upon the identification of specific objectives and the design of a properly supported system for the gathering and use of the data.

Deficiencies in reporting systems in relation to this information function are well known. The problems of relating the information derived from health services reporting to the prevailing disease pattern and to the coverage that the health services provide are not easily overcome. However, properly designed and supported data systems at this level of simplicity can be incorporated into CHW programmes. For example, in Haiti CHWs gathered data that was used in monitoring and redirecting the thrust of the programme (Berggren *et al.* 1981). This surveillance system led to priority being given to issues that reflected true needs rather than the predelictions of the providers of health care.

Any data-gathering concerning disease surveillance or assessment of work-load must be supported by an adequate system for its analysis, which will derive timely and usable findings. It is also essential that analysis of the data collected should lead to feedback to the CHWs who collect them. Activities can then be directed towards identified priorities. Such feedback also confirms to health workers the value of submitting the information and might avoid the situation reported by Coyle, Davey Smith, and Sandiford in Nicaragua (pp. 220–40), where information-collecting duties were regarded as 'irksome' by the *brigadistas*.

The third function of information systems is to influence the working practices of those completing the records. This can be termed their guidance function. The discussion of information systems tends to concentrate on their functions in monitoring the performance of CHWs and their value in monitoring vital events. These may be the prime justification of the various costs of maintaining an information system, but the guidance function may be equally valuable as a further means of bridging the separation of the centre from the periphery.

The potential of this function of medical records is currently not realized in any systematic fashion. An evaluation in Papua New Guinea indicates that the effects of this influence of medical records are largely unintended and in some instances detrimental (Frankel 1982). Given the structural problem of guiding the performance of isolated staff, this guidance function of record-keeping offers an important opportunity for focusing the efforts of these workers constructively.

As Weed points out, 'the structured, problem-orientated medical record provides a focus for constructive action' (1968). A relatively sophisticated use of this approach is described by Storms (1979) of the US Public Health Service, in relation to the Indian Health Service, where clinical protocols guided auxiliaries through the problem-solving process. These protocols were subsequently examined by a supervisor to assess auxiliaries' clinical decisions and management. Systems of such complexity would be inappropriate for most CHW programmes. The guidance function of reporting systems for CHWs should not just be limited to clinical activities. However, appropriate simplified record forms can offer the same potential in CHW programmes. The particular content of such forms will depend upon the priorities in each programme and the level of education of CHWs. The use of flow charts to assist in clinical management and identification of priorities for CHWs is described by Essex (1980). Even if it does not seem practicable to introduce such a system, it is necessary at the very least to scrutinize any record forms that are used, lest they should offer unintended or undesirable influences on CHWs' priorities.

An efficient reporting system provides a key link between the periphery and the centre. Appropriate and timely data can provide an indication of the effectiveness of a programme, and suggest modifications where targets are not being met. It provides the only consistent means for programme managers to monitor events at the periphery. Through its guidance function it may also provide a major influence on the way that CHWs and their supervisors carry out their tasks. For these reasons the design and support of information systems are key tasks in effective CHW programmes.

Referral arrangements

One rationale for the employment of CHWs concerns the economics of curative medicine. Where resources are limited it is not cost-effective for treatments to be given higher in the referral hierarchy when they could equally successfully be given at a lower level. In addition, CHWs' ability to treat potentially fatal illness is an important contribution to the welfare of populations otherwise denied ready access to health services. However, their clinical repertoire is necessarily limited, even where they are allowed to administer injections. Therefore these two aspects of CHWs' curative role can only contribute to an equitable and complete service where their activities are complemented by an adequate referral system.

This may be well recognized in China (Huang 1988), but elsewhere referral systems are commonly poor or non-functioning (England 1978; Storms 1979). There are a number of reasons for this. Physical distance is often an important barrier to successful referral. In such circumstances CHWs should be trained and equipped to manage a wider range of conditions than might otherwise be the case. Cost, social distance, a poor opinion of the health centre, domestic or other commitments, may be as important in discouraging referral as physical distance. A case study of an Indonesian project described the problem with referral that arose from the lack of co-operation from hospital staff. It seemed . . . 'as though hospital staff regarded the . . . [CHWs] . . . as rivals in the health "business"' (Williams and Satoto 1983).

Levels of referral in CHW programmes are rarely stated. In the Narangwal nutrition study 90 per cent of patient contacts were reported as being handled capably by CHWs, implying a referral rate of 10 per cent (Kielmann *et al*. 1978). This figure would not be representative of routine CHW referral, as in this project each CHW was supported by weekly visits from a doctor and a public health nurse. In these circumstances referral did not require the patient to leave the village. In one district in Papua New Guinea, some 2 per cent of patients were referred to the health centre by aid post orderlies (Frankel 1984). Aid post orderlies (APOs) were permitted a wider range of treatments than many CHWs, including penicillin injections. A likely general rate where referral might be indicated is probably somewhere between these two figures. The rate of those successfully referred will depend upon the strength of the barriers to referral that have been mentioned. In the Papua New Guinea example, some one-third openly refused to go to the health centre.

In relation to CHW performance, the opportunity for successful referral is an important component of his or her own clinical repertoire. Links between the community and the health centre, mediated by the support group and supervisors, may help to increase successful referral, which can also represent an educational opportunity (WHO 1987). A minimal requirement is therefore that literate CHWs should receive referral letters when their patients are discharged.

The supply system

Problems in the regular supply of drugs and general supplies to CHWs are widely reported. In Tanzania, Heggenhougen and Magari (pp. 156–77) report that fewer than one-third of the CHWs evaluated had drugs other than aspirin, chloroquin, or sulphodimidine. General shortages throughout the health system are likely to be felt first at the periphery as health centres become reluctant to redistribute scarce items. The periphery is largely invisible to the centre, therefore a CHW with no medicines presents a less pressing problem to managers than an empty hospital or health-centre pharmacy.

Such general shortages may stem from a variety of causes, such as a shortage of foreign exchange or deficiencies in management systems for procuring, storing, and distribution. An important consideration here is that the materials selected should be appropriate. Criteria for appropriateness include simplicity, availability, a cost sufficiently low to be borne by the community, safety, effectiveness, and acceptability to the community (WHO 1980).

This is a major problem for central planning in that management and logistic systems can barely cope with existing demands. The considerable extension that wide dissemination of medicines through CHWs would imply could not be supported within existing economic and managerial circumstances. Problems that can arise when CHW demands are simply added to the existing supply system are illustrated in the Ecuadorian example cited by Reid *et al.* (1986).

Securing an adequate supply system is a matter of critical importance for establishing effective CHW programmes. The curative role of CHWs is in most countries one of their key functions. In addition to the integral value of treating major life-threatening and discomforting ailments, effective curative services offer an entry point to wider elements of health care, such as health promotion, and drug supply shortages can lead to a loss of faith in CHWs themselves (Walt 1990). This has been a major problem in Tanzania (pp. 156–77), where frustration has set in due to the inability to provide competent curative services because of drug shortages. Much of the poor effectiveness revealed in evaluations can be attributed to this conflict.

It may therefore be counterproductive to mobilize CHWs where basic supplies will subsequently be quite inadequate. The CHW in such circumstances would be likely to become discouraged, and it would be difficult to develop subsequent support for a programme that begins inauspiciously. This has been the experience in many countries. For example, Sudan and Ethiopia reported distribution problems which led to a failure to offer a continuous service, and hence a lessening of confidence in the programme (WHO 1980). A strong case could therefore be made for precedence being given to the design and support of the supply system as one component of relations between the centre and periphery, before the wide deployment of CHWs is contemplated.

Intersectoral co-operation

Fundamental health improvement can only come about through broad-based changes mediated by activities straddling a number of sectors. It was considered particularly vital in war-torn Nicaragua (pp. 220–40), where mass organizations were used both to overthrow the Somoza regime and in subsequent reconstruction. In practice, the integration of health services with other sectors is usually poor. The health sector in most countries is characterized by a relatively popular curative service, preventive activities of varying penetration, and a struggling promotive programme that may have more coherence on paper than on the ground. However, the fact that such programmes may gain limited support and a limited response does not imply that people are indifferent to health, or the sort of changes that are known to facilitate health improvements.

Part of the problem lies in the health sector itself, in that health professionals tend to favour curative activities, as was the case with AFYA staff in Tanzania, who wanted the CHWs to be a permanent cadre (pp. 156–77). However, the values and expectations of the populations served are also important. The aspects of health improvement sponsored within the health sector clearly have a limited appeal. One response to this conclusion is to reconsider the nature of promotive activities in order to increase their potential for popular support. Another response is to extend the range of influence of the health sector to encompass activities that are known to offer potential in health improvements, as well as in encouraging community support. Berman (pp. 62–87) reminds us that CHWs in Indonesia are often regarded as a prime example of 'social mobilization', but points out that this is only within the somewhat 'proscribed boundaries' of health, rather than other socio-economic determinants.

There are therefore two aspects to the issue which make intersectoral co-operation important. The first concerns the wider influences upon PHC. The second is an organizational issue, in that activities within the traditional health sector do not readily translate into concerted community action. Community participation may only take root in relation to other sectors, when health issues are regarded as more than narrowly defined concerns for curative and preventive medicine.

Findings in the WHO interregional study indicate that existing or planned support groups are concerned with wider issues than simply the support of the CHW (WHO 1984). Desai's whole emphasis (pp. 125–55) is on the need to promote self-determination and self-reliance in rural Indian communities, since to develop health is to develop people—socially, economically, and psychologically. One of Kendall's main conclusions from Honduras (pp. 241–60) is that the success of Aqua Fresca is not so much the success of the Ministry of Health programme as that of the village itself.

In a number of countries the support group is a subgroup of the village council. In others it is a specially formed group concerned with health matters. The relative effectiveness of support groups, in relation to the breadth of their interests outside the traditional health field, would be an important basis for recommendations on the most effective means of organizing CHW programmes.

Ofosu-Amaah (1983) notes that intersectoral co-operation has occurred in numerous pilot projects, but such integration seems to break down when implementation is attempted at a more general level. Walt (1990) observed that CHWs seldom establish links with other extension agents working in their community or with community organizations, or with traditional health practitioners. The important variables underlying this observation cannot concern the communities served, for their dynamics are little altered whether they are participating in a pilot project or a national programme. Instead, barriers to intersectoral co-operation must lie in the administrative structures of relevant government departments and agencies, and in individuals' professional aspirations and rivalries.

The Yaoundé Conference stressed that failures in intersectoral co-operation at the peripheral level could not be attributed to any inadequacies on the part of CHWs themselves. Without intersectoral co-operation at the national, district, and other levels, and support from these levels for CHWs and other peripheral workers, multisectoral activities cannot be expected to succeed. Failures in intersectoral co-operation often stem from traditional divisions of labour between the relevant government departments. Bureaucratic rivalry for control was one of the most significant negative features in Zimbabwe's government programme (pp. 178–219) and the struggle for power and control of the new cadre marred Nepal's earlier Community Health Leader project (pp. 102–24). One response to this problem is to broaden the organization of health care at the national level. In India, for example, a new ministry termed the Ministry for Human Resource Development, was formed to combine health with education, sports, youth, and culture, and initiate intersectoral co-operation at the highest level (WHO 1987).

These are fundamental problems which can only be tackled through national initiatives to redirect institutional forms and attitudes, but one point of departure could be to foster the common end-point of intersectoral co-operation. A strong community organization can supply the integration that may be lacking between different sectors. There are strong arguments for directing health workers' energies towards the support of community organizations, on the grounds of the ends sought by the health sector and of the means that may contribute towards securing them, which have the development of effective CHW services as only one function among a broad range of health-related activities.

KEY CHOICES IN CHW PROGRAMMES

Community health workers' functions

Implicit in the identification of the CHW according to the aims of the Alma-Ata Declaration, is the expectation that the CHW will function at the level of the community within the general areas identified as elements of PHC (WHO 1978*a*). These are summarized as education concerning prevailing health problems and the methods of preventing and controlling them; promotion of food supply and proper nutrition; an adequate supply of safe water and basic sanitation; maternal and child health care, including family planning; immunization against the major infectious diseases; prevention and control of locally endemic diseases; appropriate treatment of common diseases and injuries; and the provision of essential drugs.

This broad remit, essential to improving health status within communities, is laid at the door of the CHW, whose job description may tend to comprise almost all aspects of a comprehensive PHC programme and was certainly regarded as far too broad and demanding in Zimbabwe (pp. 178–219).

The eleven countries of the WHO interregional Study on CHWs (WHO 1984) showed striking agreement on what functions CHWs are expected to perform (Table 1.1).

More recent studies also indicate a wide range of responsibilities for CHWs in Ecuador, for example (Mangelsdorf 1988), and in Botswana, Colombia, and Sri Lanka (Walt 1990).

There is thus little disagreement about what would be desirable as CHW tasks. The ideal in broad terms is for the CHW to be effective in prevention, promotion, and aspects of development work that may ameliorate the conditions which set high levels of mortality and morbidity. It was the lack of interest in, and indifference to, prevention, promotion, and rehabilitation which has so outraged Desai in the Indian Rural Health Scheme (pp. 126–37). However, the successful execution of many of these tasks requires a considerable level of technical ability, motivation, and educational skill. Highly trained and experienced professionals would admit

Table 1.1 Tasks expected of CHWs in the WHO interregional study on CHWs (WHO 1984)

Designated tasks in all 11 countries	
First aid, treat accidents and simple illness	Immunization motivation, assistance during clinic
Dispense drugs	Environmental sanitation, personal hygiene, motivation
Pre-, post-natal advice, motivation	Refer difficult cases to health centre or hospital
Child-care advice, motivation	Maintain records, reports
Nutrition motivation, demonstration	Participate in community meetings
Designated tasks in 10 out of 11 countries	
Family planning motivation	Communicable disease follow-up, motivation of confirmed cases
Communicable disease screening, referral, prevention, motivation	Visit homes on a regular basis
Designated tasks in 8 out of 11 countries	
Nutrition action	Perform tasks outside health sector
Collect vital statisitcs	
Designated tasks in fewer than 8 countries	
Communicable disease action (7 countries)	Immunization—give shots (3 countries)
Family planning—distribute supplies (6 countries)	Perform school health activities regularly (3 countries)
Assist health centre clinic activities (5 countries)	Deliver babies (2 countries)

doubts about their ability to perform effectively in all these areas. It is therefore essential to assess the level of performance of CHWs in many of these tasks. Only with such information will it be possible to review both the training and expectations of CHWs. The cause of PHC will not be advanced by erroneous expectations of what briefly trained CHWs may achieve, but so far there have been few studies of the expectations of either the CHWs themselves or the communities they serve (Walt 1990). The WHO Study Group on Community Health Workers (1989) considered it 'unreasonable and unrealistic' to assign a wide range of functions routinely to CHWs, and recommended that governments should define functions 'according to what is practicable in local circumstances'.

There is some evidence that CHWs can be guided to perform exclusively preventive activities. For example, the 'Programme to Improve Family Nutrition' (UPGK) in Indonesia tackled prevention and promotion, primarily in relation to child and maternal nutrition, through the mobilization of village volunteers. Berman (1984) indicates that they succeeded in reaching the poorer households in the areas where they were active, and updates the results in his chapter (pp. 62–87).

Many question the value of exclusively promotional or educational activities by CHWs, since only very small behavioural changes are generally possible among their target populations (Walt 1990). However, CHWs can undoubtedly be effective in preventive programmes. For example, in one project in Haiti, mortality rates fell to one-quarter of national estimates. The bulk of the prevented deaths were those from tetanus, malnutrition, diarrhoea, and tuberculosis, and it was argued that most of the improvement could be attributed to the preventive rather than curative services (Berggren *et al.* 1981). Also in the Caribbean, a project depending largely upon nutritional intervention by CHWs resulted in the halving of under-5s mortality rates though the prevalence of malnutrition did not change (Alderman *et al.* 1973). In an Indonesian programme, the activities of volunteer CHWs concentrating largely upon preventive activities, were associated, among other benefits, with a halving of infant mortality (Haliman and Williams 1983).

These reports confirm that CHWs are capable of performing the preventive activities which dominate in their job descriptions, and that such activities can indeed produce the benefits so urgently sought in many countries. However, the general picture from CHW programmes reveals that the bias towards preventive work, which characterizes the literature, is extremely rare in practice. This fact was remarked on in the WHO interregional study, where it was noted that CHWs 'do spend at least part—if not most—of their working time seeing patients and giving (or selling) drugs' (WHO 1984).

An important model for the desirable preventive role of CHWs came from reports on China's barefoot doctors. However, reality does not always conform to the model. An evaluation of barefoot doctor activities in Shanghai County showed that only a small proportion of their working time was actually devoted to preventive and promotive work (Gong and Chao 1982). Kan (pp. 88–101) cites the decrease in Chinese VHWs' preventive work as one of the critical issues facing the future development of the programme in China today.

The job descriptions of Papua New Guinea's APOs stress their wider role, but in practice they devote themselves almost exclusively to curative medicine (Frankel 1984). In El Salvador, many village health workers thought that community education was probably more important for health, but got most satisfaction from their own dispensing activities (Capps and Crane 1989). Jacobson *et al.* (1987) were convinced that CHWs in Kenya could carry out limited curative functions without detriment to their preventive efforts, but noted that those workers who were rewarded by tokens from their communities tended to do more curative work than those who were purely volunteers.

These examples, like many others, indicate that CHWs' current contribution is largely limited to treating existing illness. Strategies for changing this bias towards cure are clearly of fundamental importance if CHWs are to achieve effectiveness in relation to the dominant influences upon health status. However, before considering how this might be achieved it is worth considering the place of curative treatments within CHW programmes.

One way of assessing the success of a health programme is by means of the measurable changes occurring in health status. Health status improved in Europe through generalized changes in the environment following the social changes resulting from industrialization. Analogies between these changes and the likely impact of development upon health status in the less developed countries are properly drawn. However, the comparability between these historical periods is limited by the changing availability of effective treatments. There are now a number of simple remedies which, if deployed competently, can be expected to produce significant improvements in levels of disease. In addition to the specific effects of certain treatments, it is plausible that symptomatic treatments can help to reduce the stresses upon young children which contribute to the cycle of malnutrition and infection.

A second reason for not denigrating curative activities is the strongly felt need for such treatments within communities which otherwise have limited access to modern therapies. Heggenhougen and Magari (pp. 156–77) confirm that Tanzanian villagers, although having no clear perceptions of the job description of their CHWs, were obviously mainly interested in curative services, and expressed a strong desire for them to be more sophisticated.

However, the strongest justification for investment in curative activities is that they may provide an important stage in the acceptance of the wider role of CHWs, and it is therefore proper that curative activities should form an important part of the CHWs' contribution.

Nevertheless, in countries where resources for health care are extremely limited, the expansion of this category of health worker cannot be justified in terms of the wide distribution of symptomatic treatments alone. Though it may be too simplistic to say that it is necessary to stress prevention and promotion, it is essential to ask why this task is not consistently given much weight in practice.

The balance of the training curriculum is not the explanation. Training in most programmes contains a considerable amount of material unrelated to clinical skills. For example, prevention and promotion are well represented in the training of India's CHWs, but in practice these workers function primarily as distributors of free medicines, with prevention and promotion being at best marginal activities (Jobert 1985).

Two explanations are advanced for this. First, it was the clients' expectation of what the CHW would do, so they conformed to their anticipated function. The question of clients' expectations is a very important one in setting the response to such programmes, as is well illustrated from China by Kan (pp. 88–101) and from Tanzania by Heggenhougen and Magari (pp. 156–77). In Nepal the village health workers were supposed to visit some 30 houses each day to give health education lessons and to record vital statistics about family members. As they carried no medicines and were not trained to prescribe when illness was detected, they could only recommend a visit to the health post. Some villagers referred to the VHWs disparagingly as 'wall writers', after their practice of signing the date of their visit on the wall for the benefit of future visits by their health assistant supervisors, and asked why they came at all if they could not offer even simple treatments (Justice 1983).

A second explanation for the preponderance of curative activities among India's CHWs was that they represented the key means of economic survival for the otherwise unemployed, educated young people who were often recruited (Jobert 1985).

It is thus clear that preventive and promotive activities present the greatest challenge to CHW programmes. These activities require very focused preparation and support if they are to succeed. It is significant that most of the programmes where some measurable benefit from such activities was experienced are characterized by precise task-definition. Unrealistically optimistic and unevaluated job descriptions clearly have no place. It is essential that CHWs are allocated tasks for which they have been appropriately prepared and may be expected to tackle competently and which are expected to prove effective when adequately performed. Task allocation should therefore be assigned on an individual basis, according to a sliding scale where CHWs' activities vary according to their proven competence.

This strategy was proposed by the WHO interregional study where it was suggested that

> Planners must . . . take care in defining (CHWs') tasks and functions not to overburden them, especially when their education is limited and they have had only short training. Generally, they could be given only a few tasks at first and these could be extended gradually by structured continuing education . . . With experience and in-service training, (they could) acquire the complement of skills that suit their circumstances. Training is organised to systematically extend the range of tasks they can perform and over time improve the quality of services they give. (UNICEF/WHO 1980).

A balance must be struck here between the merits of structured activities on the one hand and the potential problem of stifling initiative.

In setting priorities it is important to support consideration of the broad aims, which may assist development, with a rigorous analysis of what particular components of the disease ecology can realistically be tackled by specific interventions by CHWs in ways which may be acceptable to the populations served. The particular mix between these broad components of CHWs' potential contributions must be influenced by local circumstances. Where basic curative services are available nearly everywhere, the CHW is likely to be allocated predominantly development functions. Where these basic services are yet to be made available, then more comprehensive curative functions can be allocated in the short term.

It is a basic tenet of CHW mobilization that communities must be involved at all stages of deployment. The allocation of functions must also be a shared decision. It is a common observation that when the community is consulted their demands may be at variance with the priorities of the health system. They may stress curative services to the exclusion of prevention, or indeed, as has been noted above, they may reject CHW services in favour of other projects. A proper understanding by community members of the potential benefits of the differing components of CHW programmes is obviously a prerequisite for constructive participation in programme planning. But even with an informed community the approach taken in soliciting their priorities is very important. The term 'felt needs' is perhaps misleading. Discussing 'felt problems' rather than 'felt needs' can lead to more productive community involvement in the planning process (WHO 1987).

The debate over whether these workers should be multi-purpose or concerned with single issues is no longer relevant. If CHWs are to be the vehicles for PHC they cannot restrict their activities to single issues. However, diversity in the ideal range of the activities expected of multi-purpose workers must not lead to the tasks being left ill-defined, and the concept of a multi-purpose worker must not be equated with that of an all-purpose worker (WHO Study Group 1989). Unless tasks are defined with some precision, according to their potential impact upon health status, it is unlikely that programmes will prove effective, and it will not be possible for the community or programme supervisors to judge the quality of CHWs' performance.

Patterns of financing

Financing for CHW programmes can derive from government or from the community, or from a mixture of the two. There are two main reasons for advocating community support for CHW programmes. First, it is suggested that community support, whether through the use of volunteers or through remuneration of CHWs from community funds, may minimize the social distance between the CHW and the community. Second, the costs of CHWs' support will not fall on central health budgets.

The view that remuneration from government sources would be counter-productive is an attractive argument. The aims of effectiveness and cost-limitation, which in many areas of health policy appear incompatible, are both met. The idea that government remuneration would cause CHWs to identify, and be identified, with the government and not the community to the detriment of the programme is plausible, but its merits must be tested in relation to actual experience. Sanders (pp. 178–219) may feel that community representatives have been transformed into civil servants in Zimbabwe, but the argument can appear questionable where sophisticated urban services are provided free of charge, while rural populations must contribute towards their health care (WHO 1987).

A CHW programme may be supported by the community either through the use of volunteers, or through the community accepting some sort of financial responsibility. These options will be discussed in turn.

The option of supporting CHWs through 'fee- for-service' is held to be open to abuse, and for this reason not to be recommended (UNICEF/WHO 1980; WHO Study Group 1989). Kan (pp. 88–101) expresses grave concern that this method is now very common in China, and considers it a backward step on the way to the goal of PHC for all, as it introduces notions of the profit motive and private practice and may discourage attention to the real needs of villagers.

Volunteers

Here the labour cost of a CHW programme is born by the CHWs themselves. One of the few accounts of large groups of volunteer CHWs who are reported as being satisfied with non-financial incentives, such as increased status and self-respect, concerns the Banjarnegara PHC programme in Central Java (Haliman and Williams 1983). However, it is important to note that some one-third of the CHWs trained ceased to take an active role. More recently, Berman (pp. 62–87) concedes that Indonesia's efforts have violated most of the conventional wisdom on the feasibility and sustainability of mass voluntary action by CHWs, but points out that even volunteer-based programmes require significant levels of spending if they are to achieve high coverage, and concludes that the sustainability of current efforts will depend on strengthening resources.

Unpaid CHWs (*brigadistas*) were reported from Nicaragua, but these workers, mainly young people who function as auxiliaries rather than autonomous CHWs, appear at least partially motivated by the wish to be accepted for training as professional health workers (Scholl 1984). Coyle, Davey Smith, and Sandiford (pp. 220–40) also acknowledge the importance of volunteering to support a health campaign as a major feature of community participation in Nicaragua's efforts to recover from the effects of war.

The use of volunteers elsewhere is said to be associated with high attrition rates and low stability (UNICEF/WHO 1980), with consequent high costs of retraining. In Botswana, an early programme dependent upon volunteers had to be discontinued (UNICEF/WHO 1980). More commitment than might be expected was recently reported from volunteers in Colombia, but Walt's study (1990) raised serious questions about the quality of the care offered by the *promotoras* there, and also pointed out that the volunteers of Sri Lanka were regarded mainly as adjuncts of the public health midwives, and needed far more incentive schemes to make them stay on.

Contrasting experience from different parts of India is relevant here. While CHWs were allocated an honorarium of 50 Rs per month, the firm intention was that they should not see themselves as government employees. The government's response to incipient unionization and other demands for professional recognition was to rename the CHW scheme the Community Health Volunteer Scheme in 1979. Nevertheless, a proportion of these workers regarded their role as formal employment, and depended upon their honoraria for survival (Jobert 1985). However, a different picture emerges from the experience of Indian CHW projects sponsored by voluntary agencies (Mukhopadhyay 1983). In these programmes the satisfaction of valued community service emerged as the key return for the mainly low-caste women who were mobilized as CHWs.

The ideal model for such mobilization stems from early reports of the Chinese barefoot doctors. While some forms of political and social organization may facilitate the effective general use of volunteers, it is important to stress that this model of the altruistic CHW conformed to the reality of Chinese health care only to a limited extent. The ideal type of the barefoot doctor as reported in the early 1970s was both exhilarating in its potential, and frustrating in that such selfless dedication and harmonious support seemed far from the experience in many countries which clearly required such a category of worker. For example, Ronaghy and Solter (1974) wrote of the factionalism, nepotism, and wish for personal advance that made the transfer of the model difficult in Iran. However, it is now clear that these problems were also common to the barefoot doctors of China (Chen and Tuan 1983), where large numbers of them became dissatisfied and ceased working. The aspirations of barefoot doctors, including that for professional recognition, have subsequently been met (WHO 1987; Huang 1988).

Volunteer CHWs may have considerable potential under favourable circumstances, and especially in local projects. In El Salvador, it was considered advisable that all health promoters in a non-government scheme should be volunteers, since health care and community education activities were considered 'subversive' in the civil-war climate of the late 1980s (Capps and Crane 1989).

However, there is little evidence that the mobilization of volunteers in national CHW programmes is an effective policy. It is important to remember that in many of the countries establishing CHW programmes people are poor. In such countries, volunteer schemes should not be compared with the sort of system found in developed countries, where people with spare time and a reasonable income function as volunteers. This issue was considered at length by the Yaoundé Conference, where it was concluded that it may be . . . unreasonable, if not unfair, to expect the individual CHWs themselves to contribute the labour costs of the scheme' (WHO 1987). It is difficult to generalize on this issue, for there are clearly major differences in the time commitment of a CHW whose task it is to offer information on health issues to ten households, compared to the time required for a CHW to offer a curative and preventive service to a population of over one thousand. Nevertheless, the Yaoundé Conference reached the broad conclusion that '. . . it is reasonable to state that where a CHW has no other source of income, and the time demanded by the functions assigned represents a significant proportion of the day, then that CHW should expect some remuneration, whether in cash or kind, whether from the community, government or both' (WHO 1987).

Community funding

Here the CHW's time and medical supplies may be paid for entirely, or in part, from local funds. The viability of such schemes relates largely to the nature of the responsible local organization, and this in turn is an expression of the political system. The community support of CHWs in Ethiopia (UNICEF/WHO 1980) and China (Chen and Tuan 1983) relate to the formal nature of local institutions in those countries. Kan (pp. 88–101) devotes considerable attention to the influence of the socio-economic changes of the last decade in rural China on the system of VHWs, especially their financing. Changing from a collective co-operative economy to multiple forms of ownership, and replacing brigades by a township/village system has resulted in varied financial patterns, which are unevenly distributed. As many as 95 per cent of villages report that they now have no collective funds for training VHWs.

Where community funding is anticipated, an enduring programme is extremely unlikely to emerge in the absence of any cohesive form of support group. There are numerous examples of CHW programmes that founder through the unpredictable nature of funding of this sort (for example, Ofosu-Amaah 1983). One means of community funding which can prove reliable is through drug sales. This form of financing is widespread (WHO 1984). Some contribution from consumers towards the costs of medicines may be unavoidable in many countries, but this source of funding for CHW programmes should be questioned on general grounds. Where the long-term aim is to develop broad programmes for health improvement, the use of profits from drug sales can only reinforce the dispensing role of CHWs to the detriment of the PHC approach, and possibly to the detriment of clients where prescribing practices may not be sound.

Some sort of community support for CHW programmes offers the best hope for effective local programmes, with genuine participation and accountability, but there are almost universal problems with achieving consistent and regular payments in the context of the aspects of community involvement that have been discussed at length above.

Central support

The 1979–80 interregional study (UNICEF/WHO 1980) reported that the trend appeared to be toward payment by the government. This has 'advantages in job security and programme stability, and is to be recommended for full-time CHWs'. However, it was also pointed out that this may reduce the likelihood of the people to be served regarding the CHW as 'theirs' and hence accountable to them.

In all eleven countries of the WHO interregional study (WHO 1984) the majority of funding came from outside the community. Nevertheless, a community contribution was mentioned in a number of these countries, through drug sales or various fund-raising activites, though the percentage contribution that this may represent was not specified. This would be essential information for monitoring the relative benefits of various approaches to funding.

It therefore seems that, while the general argument for minimal central support may be attractive, in practice a lack of central funding is likely to jeopardize a programme. In Tanzania, Heggenhougen and Magari (pp. 156–77) report that a new system was introduced in 1983, but so far there has still been no government money to support it and the question of remuneration from government, community, or both is still unresolved, even though the CHWs are regarded as 'frontline health workers'.

Thus the economic argument may look different when viewed from the point of view of the community and of the CHW. Many of the most successful programmes, such as those in Costa Rica, China, and Papua New Guinea, have in fact included CHWs supported wholly or in part by central funds. Costa Rica's programme is particularly effective, and it may be relevant that 97 per cent of the resources required for extended coverage of health services come from national government, and 3 per cent from local communities (Villegas 1977).

There is no doubt that self-sufficiency and community action are essential components of health improvement. However, it would be false to imply any necessary conflict between these aims and the requirement for central funding. On the grounds of equity, it is inappropriate to expect what may be the poorest communities to sponsor their health programmes when others are not expected to do so. Also, there is a clear need to subsidize programmes that may not otherwise be demanded. Programmes supported primarily from local sources, particularly through drug sales, are likely to settle for the lowest common denominator of curative activity. Where there may be no felt need for the sorts of prevention and promotion informed by the principles of scientific medicine, it is unrealistic to expect the poor to carry the costs of the programme.

The issue of financial support for CHWs is therefore inseparable from that of organizational support. Primary health care in communities cannot depend only upon government initiatives and central financing. Local programmes can only succeed through strong local institutions. Such institutions may be seen as a precondition for an effective programme, and may be able to mobilize local financial support for CHWs. Nevertheless, the available evidence indicates that such programmes are unlikely to endure and develop on a national scale without central support, and some central financing.

An essential requirement for further understanding of this issue is the gathering of more systematic data than has so far been available concerning the relationship between the activities of CHWs, including their attrition rates, and the different strategies of payment in different countries. In China, Kan (pp. 88–101) reveals that the main reason for losing VHWs is lack of pay, while Heggenhougen and Magari (pp. 156–77) also report that lack of financial support is one of the main reasons for a high drop-out rate.

The size of the population served

The earlier interregional study (UNICEF/WHO 1980) demonstrated a wide range in catchment populations for CHWs, from 1:100 in China, for a health aide, to 1:7000 in Turkey. Over one-half of programmes reviewed in that study included CHWs responsible for populations of over 2000. It must be borne in mind that where a population of 1000 is not highly centralized, access to CHW activities is likely to be unequal. It is well known that health centre utilization is greatly affected by distance, but even small differences in distance from a CHW can influence consultation rates (Frankel 1984), making home visiting particularly important for these workers (Walt 1990).

The later interregional study (WHO 1984) showed a lower range of catchment populations. Only Jamaica and the Sudan reported over 1000, and the maximum catchment population advocated for rural CHWs was 750, with 1000 deemed acceptable for urban areas.

The question of catchment population cannot be separated from the range of duties expected of the CHW, and the anticipated time commitment. Questions of cost are also critical here, as where CHWs are supported from central funds there is a direct relationship between the costs of the programme and the designated catchment population. This issue will therefore be considered further below.

Hours of work

The competent execution of the range of tasks commonly allocated to CHWs must, unless the catchment population is very small, comprise a full-time job. The time-consuming nature of the task was described for a Costa Rican CHW (Harrison 1981) who, with a catchment population of some 2000, held three two-hour clinics each week, attempted to visit 12–16 houses each day, and was constantly on emergency call.

This Costa Rican account concerned one particular CHW, presumably selected for his level of dedication, but it was unclear whether his activities represented the norm in that country. The limited international data available concerning the actual performance of CHWs suggest that this degree of application is unusual. Papua New Guinea's APOs are also full-time CHWs. While their job descriptions include a wide variety of tasks, their activities are in practice largely limited to curative clinics. In one evaluation of their working week (Frankel 1984), it was found that they held clinics for an average of just under three hours per weekday, and were generally available for consultation on approximately one-half of all days of the study. The mean number of cases treated was 124 per week (ranging from 35 to 196) from a catchment population of approximately 1000. It is commonly remarked that CHWs do not want to be available outside whatever hours are regarded as normal working hours in the formal health sector, as, for example, in Botswana (WHO 1986*a*). The CHW in India, intended as a part-time worker, treated on average 26 persons per fortnight (Maru 1983).

It would be fruitless simply to propose that CHWs should be encouraged to do more. If they are to achieve their potential contribution towards improving health status in currently under-privileged areas, that is obvious. However, any change in their contribution can only follow the sorts of structural adjustments, including adequate central and local support, that are discussed at length above. Before assuming that CHWs do not do enough, and should do more, it is important to consider the sort of allocation of time that would be required for these workers to make a more comprehensive contribution.

There is little information available concerning the time that health workers devote to each patient or each task. The Narangwal nutrition study is interesting here, in that the project was largely implemented through CHWs, and its impact on health status was significant. One relevant set of findings from that project concerns the contact time betwen CHWs and the children in their care

(Kielmann *et al.* 1978). This amounted to some seven minutes per child per week. If we consider a CHW responsible for some 250 children, contact at this intensity would require over 20 hours per week in this component of their duties. If we add travelling time and social preliminaries, child care of a sort that the Narangwal study demonstrates can be effective, it would provide a full-time job for a CHW, to the exclusion of the variety of other preventive and clinical tasks with other age-groups that the CHW should ideally conduct.

In the Kavar project (reported in Ofosu-Amaah 1983) the CHW had a variety of functions, including simple treatments, preventive activities, record keeping, and involvement in community development activities. With a catchment population of some 500 people these tasks were said to occupy some 20 hours per week.

The inescapable conclusion of a proper consideration of the time that is required to perform the range of tasks that are generally held to be desirable is that the CHW's job is a full-time one, unless the catchment population is much smaller than is generally reported. Where CHWs are to be designated as part-time they must either serve a small catchment population or have allocated to them a limited range of functions.

Recruitment criteria

Despite vast social and cultural diversity in areas implementing CHW programmes, some clear patterns are emerging as to the relative merits of different categories of recruits.

Sex

Of the countries' programmes reported in the interregional study (WHO 1984), six had mostly male CHWs, one (Jamaica) had all female CHWs, three (Botswana, Columbia, and the Philippines) mostly female, and one (Benin) required CHWs to work in pairs, one female and the other male or female. In Zambia, 78 per cent of the 1120 trained CHWs are male (Twumasi and Freund 1985). In these countries men therefore predominate as CHWs.

Papua New Guinea's APOs are almost exclusively male, though females are now admitted for training. However, it is notable that one of the most effective APOs known to the author is a middle-aged woman. She is trusted and reliable, always available for duty, forceful, and energetic in preventive as well as curative work, indeed a model CHW. In India, while there was no formal male preference in the planning of the CHV scheme, a mere 6.3 per cent were women, though 70 per cent of users were women and children (Bose 1983). Evaluations indicated that women performed much better than men.

There may be special circumstances where men are preferable to women as CHWs; for example, in Costa Rica the amount of travelling required is said to necessitate the selection of men (Harrison 1981). Nevertheless, the bulk of the critical health issues to be addressed affect women and children primarily. While good data are not available it also appears that women may be more prepared to persevere with the task of CHW. Jamaica, with all female CHWs, reports an attrition rate of only 4 per cent (WHO 1987). Other information on attrition rates and effectiveness of CHWs of either sex would be useful here, but it does seem that, on grounds of access to the section of the population at risk and on grounds of commitment, women are in general preferable to men as CHWs.

In some countries it is now the pattern for women to be recruited in preference to men. For example, in the Philippines the Barangay health workers are predominently female, as in Philippine culture it is appropriate for women to take such a role (WHO 1987). In Ecuador, Mangelsdorf (1988) did not feel that any overall statements of suitability based on demographic characteristics were appropriate, but commented that younger, single women seemed to perform slightly better during training. Walt (1990) observed that most of the CHWs in the three countries studied (Botswana, Colombia, and Sri Lanka) were women in their 20s or 30s, and Alaskan community aides have been reported as also mainly women (Haraldson 1988). McConnell and Taylor (pp. 102–24) describe the use of women-only in the more decentralized and integrated CHV programme in Nepal, pointing out the difficulties that arise when such women can only be supervised or trained by men.

At the opposite extreme are those countries where strong barriers to female recruitment exist. However, even here the mobilization of female CHWs need not provide insuperable barriers. In Nigeria, the problem presented by purdah was partially overcome by forming a Men's Club (to educate men and change attitudes) with the express intent of establishing community acceptance for some female CHW activity (WHO 1987).

Age and education

Similar considerations apply to age and education. There is general consensus that older recruits prove to be more effective CHWs. This is to be expected in terms of the qualities relevant to CHW performance, such as social standing and a commitment to community life. This consensus is supported by the improvement in the drop-out rate in Tanzania due to the selection of more mature, married candidates (pp. 156–77).

Literacy is not an essential skill for CHWs, but in general it facilitates training. Where suitable candidates are illiterate at recruitment, essential literacy can be incorporated into the training programme (Bryant 1978). Higher levels of educational experience are certainly not necessary, though they have come to be demanded as selection criteria in a number of countries as higher levels of educational attaintment become more widespread. This requirement may have the merit that it limits the field for what is often a competitively sought position, but there is little evidence that it correlates with effectiveness or perseverance.

The relative influence of some characteristics of CHWs in a Jamaican programme was demonstrated by analysing their rates for home visits, according to selected variables (Marchione 1984). Here it was found that CHWs over 25 years of age were more energetic home visitors than younger women. In the same study, academic ability, as judged by examination scores, was inversely related to this index of effectiveness.

A formal evaluation in Papua New Guinea (Frankel 1982) showed no correlation between educational attainment and effectiveness. In the Danfa Project, it was found that the young school-leavers initially preferred as candidates proved more interested in urban employment and had high drop-out rates. Older farmers proved more stable, were preferred as opinion leaders and were interested in the work as much as in any remuneration it provided (Lamptey *et al.* 1980). In the Philippines, older candidates with lower levels of education and deeper involvement in the community proved to be the more successful CHWs (Bryant 1978; WHO 1987).

The evidence therefore suggests that youth and education in recruits are in general inversely assocaited with effectiveness (WHO

1987). Kendall (pp. 241–60) confirms this with his observations on the success of the older, more committed, locally-born Health Guardian in Aqua Fresca, Honduras.

Constructive recruitment

The key expectation of CHWs is that they should constructively influence attitudes and practices in such a way as to raise the health status of the population served. Key attributes for CHWs might therefore be social standing, a long-term commitment to the life-style of the community served, and an ability to influence, by word and example, key sections of the community, particularly mothers. It is therefore unfortunate that it has been common in many countries to recruit in practice, if not in policy, young men who may see the position more as an avenue to social advancement. Whatever benefit such recruitment offers relatively well educated young men and their families, the selection of people who are likely to aspire to other types of employment must inevitably build failure into the system.

The criteria that candidates should be of good standing in the community and that they should intend to stay there are less readily identified than their age, sex, and educational experience. These qualities are reported as formal criteria in a Kenyan programme (Storms 1979). The evaluation of a Jamaican project (Marchione 1984) found that the greater the CHWs' 'locality orientation' (more local than wider social network links), the more they visited mothers at home.

The view that a candidate put forward by the community would be the most effective recruit, is based upon the naïve view of social organization that is discussed above. In some circumstances village recruitment can work well, as reported in Alaska (Heraldson 1988), and Bolivia (Bastien 1990), but it is not uncommon for recruits to be proposed to the advantage of particular leaders, rather than in the interests of all the people who may ultimately benefit from the presence of a CHW (Ramprasad 1988; Tumwine 1989). The problem of nepotism was one of the main weaknesses of government programmes in Zimbabwe, according to Sanders (pp. 178–219), while in Nepal there were political implications and factions involved in the selection of women in the use of the traditional networks associated with the National Women's Organization (pp. 102–24).

Such practices can be seen as an expression of prevailing power relations, which may further reduce access to health care for the underprivileged. For example, it is common in Zambia for local councillors to propose their own kinsmen as candidates (Twumasi and Freund 1985). This tendency is reported almost universally (including WHO 1986*a* for Botswana, Chen and Tuan 1983 for China. A joint recruitment process which actively represents the less powerful sections of the population, in order to guard against potentially counterproductive selection practices, may be clearly desirable but politically unwelcome.

The importance of joint influence in the selection of CHWs is indicated by the Indian experience. Initially, almost all the CHWs put forward were male. When subsequent monitoring of the effectiveness of early recruits indicated that female CHWs performed in general more effectively than their male counterparts, communities were encouraged to propose female candidates. The proportion of female recruitments rose somewhat, but still comprised less than one-tenth of the total. Monitoring of performance again demonstrated the value of female CHWs. It is now proposed that all CHWs should be female (WHO 1986*a*) unless 'a suitable woman candidate is not available or not willing to work' (WHO 1984). The impact of this policy statement remains to be seen, but Desai (pp. 125–55) certainly does not feel that anything tangible has yet been achieved.

An imaginative means for recruiting appropriate candidates for CHW training is reported from Thailand (WHO 1987). The method is essentially a simplified form of network analysis. A house-to-house survey is undertaken to identify those people whose advice is most frequently sought. A village plan is drawn and each household is asked where they go for advice. Arrows are drawn on the plan towards such houses, and the house with the most arrows is likely to contain the most appropriate recruit.

The exclusion of women in most countries stems largely from their general exclusion from public office. However, the process of recruitment is also a factor. Clearly, the recruitment of mature women in India and other countries, where they are excluded on grounds other than their potential abilities as CHWs, and of mature men where there are distinct merits in mobilizing male CHWs, will require greater involvement by health personnel in local recruitment practice. This is another facet of the need for effective links between the community and the formal health sector which is one of the dominant themes of this review. The WHO Study Group (1989) stressed that acceptability to the community must be the key factor in the selection of recruits, but could not approve standardized selection criteria, since so many varying cultural, religious, and economic factors come into play. Age, sex, education, marital status, residence, and occupation must all be taken into account, but 'motivation for community service' should also be added, since 'without it a CHW cannot be successful or be accepted by the community' (WHO Study Group 1989).

Training

As with all facets of CHW programmes, training cannot be considered in isolation from the specific objectives of the programme and its continuing support and monitoring. At present it would seem that 'more time and energy have been put into developing curricula and training manuals than has ever been put into support and supervision' (Walt 1990). Also, it is essential to draw on information that is available on actual CHW performance in designing training programmes. Training is another issue which has in many cases been approached in a piecemeal fashion, guided more by immediate practical considerations than by particular educational objectives. This has been confirmed by McConnell and Taylor (pp. 102–24) when they comment on on the 12-day programme designed to train over 14 000 CHVs in Nepal.

In general terms, the working environment can be expected to influence practice more than a single training experience. The implications of influences in the working environments of CHWs are likely to direct their activities in ways that may not in general terms accord with the intended balance of their contributions. It is therefore necessary to take account of this possibility in training in order to equip CHWs with the skills which may permit them to become effective in their wider role.

Training programmes, like job descriptions, have been designed with little acknowledgement of the evidence that exists concerning current CHW performance. Where no specific evaluation has been undertaken which suggests the contrary, it should be assumed that CHWs are not performing adequately in the wider range of functions that are basic to PHC. Adjustments in training programmes can offer an important opportunity to direct CHWs' efforts more constructively. But the discussion of training must be seen in the context of the other issues that have been considered here.

Problems with training programmes for CHWs are similar to those for other categories of district health workers. These include inadequate preparation of teachers, shortage of teaching materials, and the irrelevance of much of the curricula to priority tasks and functions (Cole-King *et al.* 1979; Ramprasad 1988). In the absence of systematic evaluations of the relative effectiveness and costs of varying CHW training strategies and training materials, comments can only be based upon the descriptive material that is available.

Duration and location

The interregional study (WHO 1984) showed a marked range in the length of training, from five days to one year. In Tanzania, varying lengths of training are still reported by Heggenhougen and Magari (pp. 156–77), where it is noted 'the decision on training duration rarely derives from an estimation of the time required to train CHWs adequately to perform their job; rather, it is made on the basis of financial or personnel availability, or (perhaps most commonly) in a somewhat random manner'. The costs of training are clearly one of the support functions that must fall on central funds. With such wide variations in the duration of training it would be a comparatively straightforward task to determine the relative benefits of the different training periods. In the absence of such data, it is only possible to state that the shortest periods of training, in some cases just a few days, cannot be expected to equip CHWs with any clear conceptual framework for their role. On the other hand, it seems that extended periods at a training institute, up to a year in some cases, do not appear to result in levels of effectiveness commensurate with the investment in this component of training.

The issue of duration of training cannot be separated from that of location. It is essential to keep sight of the objectives of CHW training. The attainment of basic technical competence is clearly important, but this is perhaps the simplest objective to attain. If CHWs are to approach their wider role, they must identify with it, understand key concepts in health improvement, and be adept in convincing others of their value. Selection of suitable candidates is clearly of prime importance if CHWs are to take initiative in PHC, and it is important to foster such favourable attributes of recruits. Some training strategies, such as extended periods in an urban professional environment, could well undermine the very qualities that may characterize an effective CHW (WHO 1987). The predictable influence of inappropriate training sites is reported in the Maldives, where centralized training is said to result in limited community involvement and difficulty in relating the training experience to community needs (WHO 1986*a*).

The best solution to this problem is to site training in or near the trainees' own community, or at least an equivalent social environment. In China, one of the new policies launched by the health authorities has been to focus initial training at county centres (pp. 88–101).

Non-government organizations are often able to adopt more flexible approaches than government programmes, and their projects operate on a smaller scale. Experience in such projects may not readily be transferable to national programmes, but the training methods used for the CHWs in a programme of demonstrated effectiveness are worth considering (Berggren *et al.* 1981 for Haiti). Other features of this Haiti project, which served a population of 115 000, are also relevant in explaining its effectiveness. Supervision and support services for the 30 'auxiliaries' and 60 'community collaborators' were very strong, but the structure of training is particularly worth noting. Training was progressive, in that recruits began with employment on a daily-hire basis. They were given on-the-job training in specific tasks, and did not progress to another task until competent in the preceding one. Recruits had therefore demonstrated competence and commitment by the time they passed to full-time employment. A number of particularly proficient auxiliaries were involved in training and supervision.

Interspersing training and work experience was advocated by a number of participants in the interregional study (WHO 1984). Columbia had experience of both single-term initial training and of interspersing training with work experience (WHO 1984). Single-term training was reported as cheaper, while staggered training was more effective. Such accounts underline the urgent requirement for adequate evaluations of the various strategies for training. Where on-the-job training is not feasible, it is desirable for the training area to approximate as far as possible to the CHW's eventual working environment.

Trainers

Another facet of the common lack of a considered design in CHW programmes is that trainers are often appointed on the grounds of availability rather than suitability. Clinical skill is an important part of a CHW's competence, but such skill is also the area of competence that many recruits are most concerned to secure, and relates to the function that will be most in demand when the CHW starts work. If training is left to trainers who favour clinical skills, it is unlikely that CHWs will develop any serious identification with a wider role in PHC, particularly if the training is conducted in a clinical environment.

This was the case in Tanzania, where training took place in hospitals with an emphasis on curative medicine and didactic methods, with little practical experience (pp. 156–77). Such didactic training methods may be less appropriate than a problem-solving approach. In Ecuador, non-formal techniques were rare, with only 14 per cent of the training consisting of actual experience in the field, while over 50 per cent was formal lectures by nurses with little or no rural experience (Mangelsdorf 1988). The story-telling approach has been found to be useful, where actual occurrences, such as events surrounding the death of a child, are taken as starting points for discussion of the prevention and treatment of diarrhoea, for example.

One solution which may address this problem, as well as issues concerning supervision which are discussed below, is for training to be conducted by the same individual who will later supervise the CHW. This was the preferred arrangement proposed by the interregional study (WHO 1984). An interest in the broader issues that relate to health, as well as practical instruction in intersectoral co-operation, can be introduced by trainers and experienced workers from non-health sectors (WHO 1987).

Experienced CHWs are potentially valuable as trainers (WHO 1987). However, unless this training is performed in their own home area, they are unable to function as trainers and as CHWs. The issues raised are therefore a component of the general question concerning CHWs' careers, which is dealt with in more detail below.

Current problems concerning trainers include a lack of training skills and lack of familiarity with the realities of CHWs' working conditions (WHO 1984). These, and additional deficiencies, such as inadequate manuals and teaching materials are well known (WHO 1980, Ofosu-Amaah 1983), and can only be tackled through national programmes, where the infrastructure of trainers, manuals and support services are seen as inescapable pre-conditions for the mobilization of effective CHWs.

Career prospects for CHWs

The need to consider career prospects for CHWs is one of the clearest indications of the tension between the idealized notion of the altruistic health worker, concerned with the health of his or her community, and the aspirations of many individuals who take on this task. While every attempt must be made to minimize the disadvantages that would follow from adopting a bureaucratic model, this issue must be faced explicitly in the design of CHW programmes.

The problem has surfaced so widely that solutions to it may have almost universal relevance. The experience in India has analogies in many countries and is referred to again by Desai (pp. 125–55). The programme began in 1977, but by the following year CHWs were demanding pay and conditions equivalent to those in government service.

> The government responded by emphasising that CHWs were not government employees, but representatives of the people and social workers. They were paid only a small honorarium because their health work was only part-time. Yet the CHWs continued to agitate for higher remuneration and a recognized place in the health service itself. There were reports from different parts of the country of CHWs trying to form their own unions. The Ministry of Health rose to the occasion and in 1979 produced a curious administrative solution. They simply renamed the programme the Community Health Volunteers Scheme. The change of nomenclature from 'worker' to 'volunteer' was intended to disabuse recalcitrant CHWs of any notions that they were government employees or that they deserved anything but a modest honorarium for their work. (Bose 1983)

In China, barefoot doctors' aspirations were met in 1981 by an enhancement of pay and status for those who passed a proficiency test to give them parity with teachers. Some one-third of barefoot doctors passed the necessary proficiency test to achieve this status (Chen and Tuan 1983; Huang 1988).

In Papua New Guinea, a mixture of dissatisfaction, with a perceived indifference to their problems and specific grievances over their pay and conditions led APOs to threaten strike action. This was partially successful, particularly in relation to pay, but the broader underlying grievances concerning their lack of central support were not tackled (Frankel 1984).

There are three aspects to bridging the potential gap between the intentions of CHW programmes and the aspirations of particular CHWs. The first concerns recruitment. The selection of trainees whose characteristics are the least compatible with long-term commitment to the role of CHW is widely reported. More constructive recruitment is likely to reduce discordance between CHWs' intended role and their own aspirations.

The second relevant strategy is to support CHWs in such a way as to increase the likelihood of their being satisfied with their intended role. Means for reducing the isolation of CHWs and their uncertainty as to their contribution are discussed at length above.

The third aspect is the consideration of a possible career structure for CHWs. This can be considered either from the point of view of the health sector, or from the point of view of the individual CHW.

There are two tasks where the more experienced and able CHWs can make important contributions outside their own communities; these are supervision and training. The disadvantage of employing CHWs in these tasks is that the best CHWs may then be lost to their own communities (WHO 1984) as they become absorbed into the bureaucracy. The qualities that led to their promotion may no longer be appropriate, and they may cease to make an effective contribution. This is a common phenomenon in Papua New Guinea, where APOs promoted to supervisors often turn their backs on what they come to see as the hardships of rural life. Nevertheless, an able CHW is often the best-equipped health worker to teach and supervize, and is the least likely to offer an inappropriate role model. One means for reducing the loss to their own communities of experienced CHWs who accept these tasks is for them to operate from their home bases.

As for the aspirations of individual CHWs, a number of countries offer prospects of personal advancement. In China, the best barefoot doctors may be accepted for training as doctors (Wang 1975; Chen and Tuan 1983). Kan (pp. 88–101) confirms that those who pass are presented with 'village doctor' certificates, while those who fail become 'health aides'. In Tanzania and the Sudan, CHWs could be promoted to permanent positions in the health service (Bryant 1978). Such promotion offers an attractive prospect in countries where positions with regular salaries may be extremely difficult to obtain. However, such a career structure must inevitably bias recruitment towards those who may be less likely to persevere with the role of CHW as it is generally conceived. It may therefore be unwise to design a career structure for CHWs beyond the immediate requirements within the CHW programme itself for supervisors and trainers.

MONITORING AND EVALUATION OF CHW PROGRAMMES

Over the past century, interest in health workers of this sort has fluctuated according to impressionistic assessments of need and fashions in health policy. Through WHO initiatives, acceptance of the role of CHWs has become formalized in the health policies of a large number of countries. Health for all through CHW programmes, implies an eventual international complement of over two million such workers. However, it is striking how little is known about what CHWs actually do in relation to the tasks assigned to them, the impact of these activities upon health status, how much time they actually spend doing these various tasks, the response they find among the communities they serve, attrition rates, and costs of CHW programmes. The costs of extending this information base are minimal compared to the costs of major expansions in CHW programmes. In many instances, studies are not published, especially those presented by voluntary agencies such as in Tanzania (pp. 156–77) and this creates an additional problem of access to data.

Much of the literature concerning CHWs is exhortative only. There have been few detailed evaluations of their performance and impact (for example, Heggenhougen *et al.* 1987; Walt 1990). This gap in the literature is another manifestation of the tendency to talk about, rather than to, CHWs, and to idealize them rather than acknowledge the problems inherent in their mobilization. The dearth of reliable information on the reality of health care at the periphery is not confined to less developed countries. Information systems, and the bulk of *ad hoc* research in developed countries, also offer limited insights into such issues as the relationship between formal and informal components of health care, and the extent to which formal health care systems conform to people's own perceptions of need.

The deficiencies in monitoring and evaluation were remarked on in the WHO interregional study, where it was noted that these activities 'were not provided for in the planning of programmes; funds were not provided; reporting systems were of poor quality and ill-adapted to monitoring and evaluation purposes; those who ran the programme did not appreciate the importance of monitoring and evaluation, and those who worked in the programmes were apprehensive about the outcome of evaluation' (WHO 1980).

As so little monitoring and evaluation has been performed in national programmes, this section concentrates on future strategies for evaluation rather than past experience. There is clearly an urgent need to improve this component of existing programmes, and to make useable and comparable findings widely available.

The main issues that must be faced in the evaluation of CHWs are those that are common to all aspects of evaluation. The basic tenet in health service evaluation is that specific questions must be asked which are amenable to answer through the data that are collected. In the case of CHWs this involves setting objectives for the programme, defining satisfactory achievements, and identifying areas of study which will indicate explanations of constraints upon the programme.

The evaluation of CHWs does present some particular problems, however. They are in almost all instances, and certainly in conception, generalists with a wide range of functions. It can therefore be difficult to identify particular effects of CHWs' activities. For example, Berman (pp. 62–87) could draw 'few confident conclusions' about the impact of Indonesian CHWs on the population's health and nutrition status. Another factor to consider, as has been constantly stressed above, is that aspects of the social environment are major influences upon the effectiveness of CHW programmes. Information concerning such variables, conventionally missing from health service evaluation, must therefore be included in the evaluation and monitoring of CHW programmes.

This broader perspective is also essential in considering the outputs of such programmes. The achievement of wider benefits such as self-reliance in health care cannot be captured by measuring mortality patterns or immunization rates. If the interest in evaluation and monitoring is confined to those aspects of a programme that are amenable to the usual quantitative methods, then programmes themselves may come to concentrate exclusively upon such activities and the opportunity to learn from experience of the differing strategies for promoting PHC will be lost.

A final factor to be considered is that the CHW's role is especially critical in the less accessible parts of a country, where the logistical barriers to evaluation are likely to be even more marked and the costs even higher. This is well demonstrated in McConnell and Taylor's chapter on Nepal (pp. 102–24), a country whose geography is a 'formidable barrier to development'.

Methodologically ambitious evaluations in a number of locations can be important in refining the understanding of influences upon the effectiveness and efficiency of CHW programmes, although research funded by external agencies is not always given the highest priority by health ministers (Walt 1990). Such studies are managed by specialists, and need no further comment here, where the focus is upon evaluation and monitoring activities directed towards management decisions. The complexities of health service evaluation are perhaps exaggerated in the literature. As Cole-King (1979) says, there is 'a need to de-mystify evaluation and make it more relevant and manageable for PHC programme development'. It is important to consider the purpose of this activity. Where this is to answer basic operational questions, the requirements of evaluation and monitoring are well within the capabilities of any adequately managed CHW programme. In these circumstances, a balance must be struck between the potential management advantages of this activity and the danger of stifling programmes through over-evaluation (Bryant 1978).

Impact

An effective CHW programme might be characterized by a variety of changes in disease prevalence, life expectancy, age and disease specific mortality rates, case fatality rates, fertility rates, child growth rates, and other indices of health status, requiring varying levels of sophistication in surveillance methods.

CHW programmes can have the greatest impact in areas where infectious diseases, the diseases of poverty, are most prevalent. In these circumstances major changes in mortality rates, particularly child mortality, can be expected from an effective programme, such as in Alaska (Haraldson 1988). The greater the proportionate change in mortality that is anticipated, the cruder can be the instrument for measuring it.

Most of the countries participating in the WHO interregional study included the collection of vital statistics as a part of the CHW job description (WHO 1984). The collection of vital statistics is pointless unless it is supported by adequate facilities for processing and presenting the data for specified purposes. The following remarks are based upon the assumption that the interest in these data is to be supported by the means for processing them.

The only published measures of the impact of CHW programmes concern special projects rather than routine health service activity (for example, Haliman and Williams 1983; Berggren *et al.* 1981; Alderman *et al.* 1973; Kielmann *et al.* 1978). However, such impact assessment can be incorporated into routine programmes with relatively minor additional support to ensure that suitable data are collected systematically and then collated, analysed, and presented in an appropriate form.

For this purpose, each CHW would need to record a relatively small number of vital events, as in each population area of around 1000 people there would only be some five dozen or fewer births and deaths each year. The occurrences of births and deaths are widely broadcast in face-to-face communities, so that problems of under-reporting need not be great.

Time trends are an essential component of impact assessment. Now it would be extremely unusual for a CHW programme to be the first, or only, modern health input into an area, but it would be expected that some changes should follow its introduction or reorganization. The first task, where no reliable data already exist should be to establish baseline data. Such initial surveillance and the discussion of its findings would have the effect of sensitizing the community to the nature and purpose of the programme.

Births and deaths are categories which mean broadly the same thing to people of all cultures and levels of education, so there are no problems of interpretation in deriving mortality rates. Interpretations of disease differ, but usable disease specific mortality can also be determined to acceptable levels of validity by CHWs. The categories in the 'main list' suggested by the WHO Working Group on the lay reporting of health information (WHO 1978*b*) would be too detailed for most CHWs to use. There is no doubt that they can be used by 'barefoot epidemiologists' of similar educational experience, but the training and support requirements necessary to gain valid data could not, in most circumstances, be justified. A version of the 'minimal mortality list', simplified according to the prevailing mortality pattern and objectives of the programme, would be appropriate. Such reporting systems can be important in highlighting remediable deficiencies in a programme. For example, in the Narangwal Project, surveillance of child deaths indicated that the expected impact upon diarrhoeal and pneumonial deaths was not being achieved. Only adequate surveillance and resultant changes in standing orders produced the desired effects (McCord and Kielmann 1978).

Population denominators are more problematic, especially in areas of high migration. Where these cannot be established without an inordinate investment in demographic surveillance, the number of deaths and their probable causes still offer valuable pointers to priorities for action.

Changes in mortality have the most general application in the assessment of the impact of CHW programmes. The relevance of other effects, such as changes in nutritional status, vary according to the thrust of particular programmes, and so are not considered in further detail here.

Process

Measures of process may be used as indicators of the likely impact of a programme. For example, the percentage of families with latrines, the percentage of children immunized, or the percentage of mothers who breast-feed may offer partial guides as to the effectiveness of a programme. Process measures are also necessary for proper management of a programme.

In the context of CHW programmes the key questions concern the selection of indicators on which data can readily be collected within the structure of the reporting system, and which will allow judgements to be made as to whether the programme is meeting its objectives. A first requirement is therefore a set of clear objectives which can be expressed as specific targets. If there are no explicit objectives these will have to be determined through discussion.

Process evaluation is required at two levels. At national level, basic information is necessary to determine the effectiveness of training methods, including continuing education, to detail levels of support and supervision, and to monitor the efficiency of the medical supply network, among other issues. Attrition rates are of great relevance for national planning as well as for the wider understanding of factors that may correlate with effective CHW programmes, such as the age, sex, and educational background of recruits, the method and nature of payment, career prospects, organizational arrangements, structure of the support group and the extent of intersectoral co-operation.

At the local level, a variety of aspects of the programme are relevant. In relation to organizational arrangements, information on such issues as the frequency of support-group meetings and the number of participants, together with the frequency of supervisory visits and their content, and the frequency of continuing education, would be important.

In relation to CHWs' working activities, information on the level and equity of coverage, the performance of specified tasks in the job description, or the numbers of home visits might also be collected.

An indication of the outputs of the programme could be gained by such data as the percentage of families using a covered water supply, the percentage of mothers who received antenatal care, the percentage of children immunized to a certain level, or the percentage of children under nutritional assessment.

Formal evaluations may use the methods of social anthropology to address broader questions, such as the influence of CHWs upon peoples' choices of strategies for maintaining health or treating illness (Frankel 1984, 1986 Frankel and Lewis 1989). However, the examination of such issues cannot be confined to formal evaluations and academic studies. It is also important to focus upon certain qualitative aspects for local purposes in order to keep the broader aims of CHW programmes on the agenda, as well as to modify programmes where it is apparent that the wider objectives are unlikely to be achieved. These issues are best tackled within the context of the support group. Such involvement of the support group in the process of monitoring is an essential component of active community participation.

An imaginative means for introducing an interest in objectives to this form of participatory evaluation has been developed in Thailand. There CHWs, as well as members of support groups, are exposed to CHW programmes in villages, other than their own, where programmes are proving successful. This dissemination of the knowledge and experience gained in model villages is seen as analagous to technical co-operation at the international level, and so is referred to as Technical Cooperation among Developing Villages (TCDV). The approach was strongly endorsed for widespread use by the Yaoundé Conference (WHO 1987).

A framework for evaluation should be included in planned CHW programmes as a component of the information system. This activity should be an integral part of the programme and not conducted primarily by an outside team.

Cost

One of the assumptions upon which the interest in CHWs rests is that they are a cost-efficient means of bringing health care to the wider population. If CHWs are only supported to a limited extent from central funds, then once initial training is completed revenue costs are in general restricted to whatever supplies are issued, together with the costs of supervision and support. It is then more likely that functions otherwise performed by other sections of the health care system will be performed more cost-efficiently by CHWs. However, it is important to distinguish between efficiency and cost-limitation. While lower unit costs for each encounter may reflect greater efficiency, the wide dissemination of the service is likely to lead to raised programme costs.

In addition, most CHW programmes have failed to achieve their potential effectiveness through inadequacies in support, supervision, and continuing education. Such support services must clearly be developed within an effective CHW programme, and could be expensive in terms of staff and transport costs.

While there is little doubt that CHW programmes offer a vehicle for providing simple interventions to currently under-served populations at low unit cost, the financial implications of properly supported national programmes have not been determined. Very occasionally, attempts are made to quantify cost-effectiveness, as in a review of six CHW programmes by Berman *et al.* (1987). Berman continues with his concern for the costs and financing of CHW activities in his contribution to this book, speculating on the likelihood of the new system of *Pos Yandu* in Indonesia and its possible impact on cost-efficiency and cost-effectiveness (pp. 62–87).

For the most part, however, the absence of proper cost evaluations is a further expression of the common failure to appreciate the broad requirements of an effective CHW programme. Where CHWs are simply grafted onto existing structures they cannot be expected to have any serious impact upon health status (Ramprasad 1988; Matomora 1989). The range of support services that are essential preconditions for effective CHWs must be planned and costed. There is an urgent need to undertake such studies as part of the process of acknowledging the true requirements of effective CHW services.

NATIONAL CHW PROGRAMMES—THE WAY FORWARD?

Evidence from pilot projects leave no doubt that CHWs can be effective agents of health improvement. Little systematic information concerning the effectiveness of national programmes is available, but the evidence that exists strongly suggests that under service conditions CHWs' contributions have fallen far short of the level and range of activity which these workers must achieve, if they are to be the vehicles for widespread changes in health status. In many places they have brought symptomatic treatments to populations otherwise unserved by health services. In this they are satisfying a strongly felt need, but this contribution is only a shadow of their designated role in approaching health for all.

In a few countries, CHWs active in disease prevention and health promotion have been deployed on a wide scale, indicating that there are no insuperable barriers to their engaging in broader-based activities. Strong commitment at the political level to improving the lot of those sections of the population suffering from diseases of poverty is clearly a major advantage if CHWs are to succeed. But even in auspicious circumstances these programmes are likely to founder. Both the potential value of CHWs and the sources of their failure stem from their unique position at the interface between the health sector and the community. Where CHWs are simply grafted on to existing structures it is possible that a few remarkable individuals in favourable circumstances may make some impact, but in general the programme will fail. Effective, enduring CHW programmes on a national scale can only emerge where specific provision is made for the range of supportive activities analysed at length above.

It is therefore obvious that much of the eupohoric international response to the partial picture of China's barefoot doctors which emerged in the early 1970s was somewhat naïve. CHWs do not offer a short-term panacea. Unpaid, unsupported, and barely trained villagers cannot compensate for the failure of national health systems to offer basic services to deprived sections of their populations.

The mobilization of effective CHWs may in some instances have been jeopardized by inappropriate expectations, but this does not justify the gathering doubt as to whether CHWs have any role at all. The evidence from national CHW programmes cannot support that conclusion, and this is confirmed by the contributors to this book.

Community health *workers* have not failed. It is the CHW *programmes* that have often foundered, in that they have not offered the supportive services which are the essential precondition for an effective and enduring national programme. It is only a minor exaggeration to say that CHW programmes have not failed: they have not been attempted!

It is unrealistic to expect widespread and immediate gains from a process as complex and diffuse as the mobilization of CHWs. There may be short-term and readily measurable benefits in regions which have until now been deprived of basic health services. But the wider process of change, of which CHWs are a key component, must be approached in terms of a much longer time-scale.

That is why it is important to stand back from time to time and gather together overviews of a number of key national CHW programmes, such as those presented here.

2

Community-based health programmes in Indonesia: the challenge of supporting a national expansion

PETER BERMAN

INTRODUCTION

It is now well over a decade since Indonesia launched its first official, government-sponsored community health worker (CHW) scheme. Although Indonesia's efforts violate most of the conventional wisdom on CHW programmes, they comprise one of the largest and longest running efforts in the world.

In the last 12 years, hundreds of thousands, some estimate millions, of community health, nutrition, and family-planning workers have been trained. Most of these citizens work as volunteers, receiving no monetary compensation and often no compensation at all. They provide or participate in a fairly comprehensive package of basic services, yet they receive a bare minimum of training, preparation, and support for their tasks. In a public health system characterized by fairly low cost-efficiency, they are one of the most cost-efficient components. There are major doubts about their efficacy, but few observers feel they make no contribution to health improvement.

This chapter will review the characteristics of this mammoth system of CHWs and its programmatic and institutional background. It will focus on health and nutrition CHWs rather than the extensive system of community-based contraceptive distributors. Available information on the benefits of the programme, its shortcomings, and its cost and financing will be discussed.

Finally, it will examine the role of CHWs in Indonesia's national health system, and speculate on the challenges to be met to ensure benefits from current accomplishments.

A BRIEF HISTORY OF CHW PROGRAMMES IN INDONESIA

Today's national CHW system in Indonesia has its roots in early experiments both by the public sector and by voluntary organizations. Public action to involve villagers in community health activities can be traced to the epidemic control services of the colonial health system prior to independence. As in many countries, Indonesia has been training traditional birth attendants in modern hygienic practice for decades, trying to involve them in referral of high risk pregnancies to qualified antenatal care and supervised deliveries. Community-based intermediaries (now called 'kader') have long been used in government programmes for agricultural extension, non-formal education, and other activities (Judd 1987).

A more immediate impetus for the current programmes came from innovations in the voluntary sector. Perhaps best-known were projects in Central Java and Yogyakarta which demonstrated the feasibility of volunteer CHWs carrying out a wide range of tasks, including simple curative care, growth monitoring, managing community-based health insurance and supplementary feeding. This process, with its achievements, trials and errors, is inspiringly described in Johnston (1983) and Suyadi *et al.* (1977). The innovators paved the way for greater efforts and also developed the initial technical inputs for programmes, such as training curricula and growth charts, much of which is still in use in national programmes today.

Along with these experiments, the government was also gaining experience and interest in the potential for community-based action. This included the use, by the National Family Planning Coordinating Board, of community-based contraceptive distribution posts to improve access to contraceptive supplies, and early efforts to train community-nutrition workers through the Applied Nutrition Programme. In recognition of these developments, the Ministry of Health finally undertook a formal pilot project to develop CHWs in one regency in Central Java (Waloeyo 1976), and began expanding a community-based nutrition programme emphasizing growth monitoring by 'mothers as health workers' (Rohde and Northrup 1977).

Although some argued that the 'good idea' which CHW programmes represented still needed further development and experimentation, by the time of the 1978 International Conference on Primary Health Care in Alma-Ata (WHO 1978*a*), a public policy steamroller was in motion. Within a few years, numerous government departments and national programmes enlisted volunteer community workers (all referred to as kaders) and trained them briefly in health and nutrition related activities. Foremost in this group was the national family-planning programme, which retooled its community-based contraceptive distribution posts to include growth-monitoring and nutrition education, (for a more detailed description of this process, see Rohde and Hendrata 1983).

However, family planning was not the only scheme. Within the Ministry of Health, two national kader schemes were expanding rapidly; one was a nutrition programme, the other a community health development programme. Other programmes training community-based workers to do health and nutrition activities included a national effort to enhance the role of women in development, sponsored through a new Minister for Women's Affairs, and parallel efforts to stimulate youth group activities for development, sponsored by a new Minister for Youth Affairs. International donors, including UNICEF, the World Bank, WHO and USAID, eagerly supported these efforts.

While doing field work in 1981, Berman found numerous villages in which up to six different government programmes had introduced community-based health or nutrition actions, and trained kaders since the mid-1970s. Obviously, there was a great deal of overlapping and replication among these schemes. In general, the same CHWs were often trained several times by different programmes and bore an added unnecessary burden of time spent in training and paperwork in reporting to several different departments (Judd 1987).

Much of this activity was not well-conceived or supported. Most of these different schemes faded from the scene or were allowed to merge into the more persistent efforts promoted by the Ministries of Health and the National Family Planning Coordinating Board, both of which tended to take a leading role in interdepartmental efforts in this area anyway.

More recently, there has been a major effort to consolidate the different health and nutrition kader schemes with the principal government role reverting to the Ministry of Health. The unifying concept has been the Integrated Service Post (*Pos Yandu*), which is a location, in the community, at which monthly growth-monitoring sessions are organized by CHWs, sometimes augmented by supplementary feeding. These sessions also become an opportunity for attendance by government health, nutrition, and family-planning workers, who provide a range of services, with priority given to the following functions: immunization, diarrhoeal disease control, antenatal care, health and nutrition education, and family planning. It is hoped that this combined approach will reduce the confusion engendered by so many different efforts in the past as well as strengthen the link between the government's extension personnel and the community efforts. Formal linkage with specific preventive services, such as immunization, is also expected to improve the effectiveness of community-based activities, which in the past were almost exclusively educational.

Throughout these periods of programmatic diversity and then consolidation, the absolute scale of CHW activities in Indonesia has expanded dramatically. By September 1988, UNICEF reported that about 50 000 villages, or 86 per cent of all villages in Indonesia, had approximately 200 000 weighing posts covering 81 per cent of all children under five (Government of Indonesia and UNICEF 1988). This is unequivocally an impressive achievement.

WHAT KIND OF CHW HAS INDONESIA DEVELOPED?

The term CHW, while widely used around the world, represents a diverse range of intentions and experiences in PHC (WHO 1987*b*; Walt 1988*b*). This diversity extends to several important dimensions: the skills and training of CHWs, the extent to which they represent the community (or parts of the community) or the formal health services, and their role as 'lackey or liberator' (Werner 1977). A chronology of government programmes, and quotes from official documents, does not represent adequately the meaning or significance of CHWs in the context of community life or the health system.

To make matters more complex, the characterization of CHW activities is often determined in large part by the biases and expectations of observers, as well as by the purpose of their observations. If CHWs are not active 'liberators' (in the sense of significantly transforming the way villagers interact with modern medicine or, even more demanding, State power) is their effort then somehow inadequate or not authentic? If they foster only changes in knowledge or attitudes regarding health problems, outcomes to which it is hard to give epidemiological significance, are programmes not effective? Conversely, should the claims of programme promoters, possibly exaggerating the impact of social mobilization on health status, be accepted as fact? If communities participate enthusiastically in activities which have little clinical benefit, should one accept it as success?

In describing real programmes, especially very large-scale ones supported by governments, the nature of CHW activities may be far from ideal on many dimensions, yet still (subjectively) judged to be significant. Is the glass half-full or half-empty? Ultimately, analysts must make their own decision, but it is important to be frank about what has been accomplished, what still needs to be done, and what has not been attempted.

The lackey or liberator dichotomy proposed by Werner refers to the role of CHWs as a force for social change, in such aspects as giving voice to the needs and demands of villagers to the State, or developing greater self-reliance or less dependence. CHWs in Indonesia have been cited by UNICEF as a prime example of 'social mobilization' for health. Yet one must acknowledge that, within the current political context in Indonesia, the extent to which CHWs mobilize social action is within fairly proscribed boundaries. They are usually selected by the village elite, who are often closely allied with the ruling regime. CHWs are usually people affiliated in some way to this elite, with a common interest in satisfying the demands of government health functionaries for meeting targets (Judd 1987). They face sanctions and loss of support if they step beyond the acceptable limits of community action or politics (William and Satoto 1983). If they 'liberate' it is with a soft voice and without challenging the existing power structure. They touch on issues of health knowledge, attitudes, and behaviour, not their underlying socio-economic determinants.

Within those limits, CHWs in Indonesia have helped mobilize an impressive level of community action for health improvement. Millions of mothers and children turn out monthly to attend village growth-monitoring sessions. Evaluations have reported very high levels of awareness of key programme messages concerning the importance of growth for health, and the link between proper child feeding, nutrition, and growth. All of this community action is voluntary, including the significant time contributions of the CHWs themselves. While not all CHWs show great dedication or enthusiasm for these activities, throughout the country one can find kaders who have contributed consistently for years to the maintenance of routine health action in their neighbourhoods.

Another important dimension of Indonesia's CHW programmes relates to the level of training and skills imparted to CHWs, and their capacity for independent action. The early CHW projects developed by voluntary organizations tended to provide CHWs with enough training to enable them to act as front-line service providers, under the supervision of medical or paramedical staff from the health centre. This included provision of a drug kit and instruction on therapy for common illness. Training was continuous, as new skills and activities were added. The emphasis was more on CHWs as *practitioners*.

As CHWs were integrated into government programmes, they were limited much more to the role of health and nutrition *promoter*. Training for new CHWs is for one week or less, hardly enough time to acquire much in the way of skills or understanding. In-service training is sporadic and limited. Initially, some government programmes provided CHWs with a drug kit, but this usually contained only over-the-counter supplies that were widely available in village shops. Today, CHW supplies are mainly oral rehydration salts (ORS), Vitamin A capsules, and iron folate tablets. Their main tasks are to organize village growth monitoring sessions, weigh children and maintain growth charts, and advise mothers on proper care in pregnancy, lactation, and growth maintenance. These are clearly primarily promoter functions. There has been concern for some years that CHWs are not well prepared to advise and counsel mothers, thus weakening that crucial function.

These are the choices that Indonesia has made in developing a national CHW programme. They are significant in their effect on programme impact and on the nature of community-based activity. The programme has lacked substance in terms of clinical interventions, although recent changes may provide a remedy. It is not an active force for direct social change, although it may be affecting health behaviour in important ways. Yet national commitment to this indigenous concept of kader remains, and the programme is a

Table 2.1 Expansion of kader programmes and *Pos Yandu* in Indonesia*

Year	Number of CHW villages	Number of Pos Yandu	% of villages included	% of under-5s with access
1979	1 700	Pre-PY	<5	
1984	31 000	Pre-PY	About 50	
1986	38 000	124 000	57	51
1987		134 000		60
1988 (projected)	50 000	199 000	>80	81
1989 (projected)		217 000		89
1990 (projected)	60 000+	245 000	100	100

* Sources: UNICEF-Jakarta 1986; Government of Indonesia and UNICEF 1988.

significant component of the country's health system. This major national programme, using volunteer workers, stands up as a challenge to the conventional wisdom that such mass voluntary action is neither feasible nor sustainable.

RESULTS OF INDONESIA'S CHW PROGRAMME

Numbers

In the world's fifth most populous country, spread out over 3000 inhabited islands, any nation-wide effort faces difficulties of scale and expansion. One sure sign of Indonesia's accomplishments with community-based health action is its achievement of 86 per cent coverage of all villages with kaders in a little over a decade. Table 2.1 presents some figures on the expansion of CHW activities in villages from the late 1970s onwards.

Maintenance

Dependence on voluntary action in the community has been judged by many to be not feasible. Once accepted as feasible, critics expect it not to be sustainable. Volunteer CHWs may begin with high enthusiasm, but their commitment is said to wane and as this happens community activities cease (Walt 1988*b*).

This problem has plagued health kader efforts in Indonesia, but not overwhelmed them. Studies estimate annual drop-out rates of 20 per cent or more, giving the average kader a work-life of three to five years (Berman 1985). Since kaders are trained at the rate of about one for each 10–20 families, there are often other kaders in the same hamlets or villages who remain active and maintain village activities. Periodically, replacements for those who drop out are selected. Often these replacements are not formally trained, they simply learn from their companions. For villages receiving frequent input from health centre staff, it may be possible to maintain programme activities. For those getting less input, kader drop-outs lead to a steady degradation of activities, first in terms of quality and ultimately in terms of frequency and participation. Despite the low budgetary cost of using volunteer kaders, there is still a real cost in terms of wasted training and decline of activities after investments have been made. Judd (1987) and others have noted that there are often one or two kaders per village who do most of the work and tend to stick with the programme. They have related this to possible obligations of these individuals to the village administration, although they are often honestly committed to programme goals as well. Studies have shown that kaders work about 8–10 hours monthly and that they may receive informal remuneration, such as free treatment at health centres. Thus working as a kader has some rewards and may not be overly demanding on villagers who do not face substantial opportunity costs from the loss of a small amount of time each month: for example, housewives in better-off families. This may account for why so many kaders keep working, and despite 'drop-outs' activities continue in many villages. Unfortunately, because recruitment and training of replacements is often omitted or delayed, the quality of service may be poor. This is an important shortfall resulting from the dependence of community activities on government resources.

Coverage

The total numbers of CHWs trained and *Pos Yandu* created are more indicators of accessibility of services, rather than the extent to which the population is reached by real health activities in the community.

Table 2.2 Results of national *SKDN** monitoring system, 1987

Total number of children enumerated	19.5 million
Percentage of all children contacted (K/S)	76%
Percentage of all contacted children weighed (D/K)	80%
Percentage of all weighed children gaining weight (D/S)	61%
Percentage of under-5s with contact with well-child services, 1982†	11%

* Source: Government of Indonesia and UNICEF 1988.
† Source: Biro Pusat Statistik 1982.

Coverage of children in the target age-group (0–5) has been studied in several major programme evaluations, as well as numerous smaller studies. It is also a major part of the built-in monitoring of the programme.

The monitoring system is designed to combine needed feedback to the community, in a form they can comprehend and use, with reporting to the formal health services. It has been based on the initials *SKDN*, representing the Indonesian words for 'all', 'growth charts', 'weighed', and 'gained weight'. The total number of *all* target age-group children in the community should be known. From this, the number of *growth charts* distributed for children represents those children ever-reached by activities. The monthly calculation of the number of children *weighed* allows calculation of the most recent coverage, using a proportion. The number who *gained weight* is a simple indicator of nutritional welfare. By calculating proportions such as (*K*/*S*), (*D*/*K*), (*N*/*D*), and so on, communities can measure and track their own progress. A colourful wall-chart has been provided for the village weighing post for this purpose. An ideal community programme will succeed in having all indicators equal to *S*; that is, all children reached, participating, and gaining weight every month.

The results of the official *SKDN* monitoring system for 1987 are shown in Table 2.2. The average percentage of all children in the target age-group who have had any contact with the programme (*K*/*S*) is 76 per cent. As one would expect, there is considerable variation in (*K*/*S*) throughout the country, ranging from 40 to 100 per cent.

Attendance at weighings for those children registered by community workers (*D*/*K*) is reported to average 80 per cent. If one calculates true coverage with weighing (*D*/*S*), the average is 61 per cent. To give some perspective to these figures, one should note that a recent estimate of the percentage of target-age children using clinic-based well-being and well-child services is 11 per cent (Biro Pusat Statistik 1982).

Assessing programme coverage solely in terms of *SKDN* may be misleading. Much depends on accurate determination of the total target population (*S*). There is evidence that community workers are often not very thorough in enumerating children at the beginning of programme activities. This denominator must also be constantly revised, as new children are born and older children 'graduate' from the target age-group. This can be seen in well-run programme villages, but not all meet this standard. There is also confusion sometimes about the actual area to be covered. Programme activities may be initiated in one or two hamlets in a village, whereas the total population of 0–5s reported is for the village as a whole. In such cases true coverage is underestimated.

The reported coverage levels, and the problems with the *SKDN* system certainly indicate that some children, and in certain areas many children, are not being reached. Who tends to be left out and what are their characteristics in relation to programme objectives? For example, does the programme tend to reach more, or less, of the undernourished and the poor? Since national data show less than two per cent of under-5s as severely malnourished, and approximately another one-third having some signs of undernutrition, even relatively good coverage could be missing most of those in need (Centre for Nutrition Research and Development 1982). When participation occurs, is it regular or sporadic? Some answers to these questions are available from large programme evaluations, as well as in-depth studies of CHW communities—often selected from areas with higher coverage. Table 2.3 summarizes important points from a number of these studies.

In a study of seven villages selected for excellent programme activity, Fajans and Sudiman (1983) reviewed kader records and reported coverage with weighing of all children from 48 to 96 per cent. This was not verified through a survey to determine the actual number of under-5s, but they were confident that these data were fairly accurate. There was no association between nutritional status

Table 2.3 Summary of studies assessing coverage with CHWs in Indonesia

Study authors/ Year	Location	Includes full enumeration of population	Number of villages included	% of target group ever reached by CHW	Frequency/ regularity of coverage	Characteristics of users	Comments
Centre for Nutrition Research and Development, Bogor 1982	6 provinces W. Java, C. Java, E. Java, S. Kalimantan, S. Sulawesi, N. Sumatra	N	99	40	28% weighed last month	Not known	Sample of all programme villages. May have underestimated coverage by not focusing only on programme hamlets
BKBBN *et al.* 1986	E. Java, Bali	Y	1790	70	41% reporting 'frequent' attendance	Mothers reporting attendance tended to have better nourished children	
Fajans and Sudiman 1983	Bali, W. Java, C. Java, W. Sumatra	N	7	50	Fairly high	No indication of low participation by undernourished	Focus on well-performing villages

Berman 1985	Central Java	Y	4	84	71% weighed last month	Some bias towards low income groups. Low wt for age children proportionally included
Allan and Goodwin 1987	S. Sulawesi	N	14	NA	<30% of target population on average	NA
Achadi and Berman 1988	Central Java	N	1	50	Proportion ever reached constant over 4 years. Significant decline in frequency/ regularity of attendance over time	Children with low wt/age included proportionally in participants

and programme participation, suggesting at least no bias away from higher risk children.

Berman (1985); Berman *et al.* (1989), and Achadi and Berman (1988) present data from a few villages benefiting from special attention as part of a pilot project financed by the World Bank. Average coverage with weighing, based on a total enumeration of under-5s was about 70 per cent. There was a marked bias towards the inclusion of children from lower-income groups, suggesting a focus on the more malnourished population. Achadi and Berman (1988) analysed four years of weighing records from a single village in this area. While the proportion of children reached with weighing and related services remained relatively constant over the period (at about 50 per cent), the frequency and regularity of attendance diminished steadily. However, there was no change in the distribution of nutritional status among those attending.

Although data on the distribution of weight-for-age in the population as a whole was not available, the figures suggest that the undernourished are being included in programme activities at least proportionally.

Less positive results are available from several larger surveys of CHW programme villages. A national study of kader activities in nutrition programme villages in 1982 reported 45 per cent of children in project villages had received growth cards, and 28 per cent had been weighed in the previous month (Center for Nutrition Research and Development 1982). These results did not correct for under-enumeration of kaders or for the incorrect specifications of the weighing catchment area.

A large-scale evaluation of the integrated nutrition and family planning kader programme villages in East Java and Bali, conducted by the National Family Planning Coordinating Board (BKKBN *et al.* 1986) reported that, on average, 70 per cent of mothers had attended a village weighing session, with 41 per cent reporting 'frequent' attendance. These attendance figures showed a large range across villages, for example 'ever-attended' ranged from 11 to 100 per cent in Bali, and from 15 to 100 per cent in East Java. There was evidence in East Java that mothers who reported 'ever-attending' had children with somewhat high nutritional status. This could represent programme impact or a bias in coverage. Income was also associated with nutritional status and hence, attendance. A smaller study in South Sulawesi (Allen and Goodwin 1988) reported similar low rates of overall coverage, under 30 per cent in fourteen *Pos Yandu*. However, attendance of those registered was fairly high and regular.

The sum of these studies suggests that, while high coverage with growth monitoring and other activities has been attained and sustained in many villages, these are still a minority. More typical is the situation where coverage remains relatively low for a community-based activity (under 50 per cent), and in many cases a third or less of children under five. There is a tendency for coverage to decline over time, although the effects of the stimulus of the new *Pos Yandu* model have not yet been measured. Community-based activities have been shown consistently to reach some of the lower-income groups and the undernourished, even though in many cases the majority may not participate.

Health communication and other interventions

Attendance or coverage at weighing sessions indicates whether children and mothers are being reached by programme activities. But what are they being reached with?

Indonesia's CHW programmes seek to increase awareness and knowledge concerning factors affecting child health and nutrition. The focus is on mothers and families, empowering them with appropriate tools for monitoring the health of their children and providing them with the information, motivation, and skills they need to make a difference. Even when supplementary feeding is provided for children showing low weight-for-age or poor growth, it is intended more to be educative than rehabilitative. The option of clinical treatment is kept in the background as a resort when community-based resources fail. Only more recently, with the advent of *Pos Yandu*, have health centre services been integrated into activities in the community.

The concept of the programme places most of the burden of informing, educating, and counselling mothers on the kaders, by far the most difficult of their tasks. In addition, they perform several other technical tasks, such as proper weighing and charting, and, administration/distribution of oral rehydration salts, high dosage Vitamin A capsules, and iron folate tablets.

Kaders usually receive only one week of training. Most observers of the programme have felt that this does not provide them with sufficient skills or experience to be effective one-on-one counsellors. Their repertoire is often limited to a few distinct but general programme messages: for example, weight gain measures how well your child is doing; healthy children gain weight as they get older; food intake and feeding practises are important factors affecting weight gain.

Almost all studies of the CHW programme report very high awareness of these messages. For example, in East Java and Bali, BKKBN *et al*. (1986) reported that 90 per cent of mothers knew the health significance of steady weight gain. Knowledge regarding proper weaning practices and feeding of colostrum was lower. Familiarity with the weighing message was significantly higher than attendance at weighing sessions. Fajans and Sudiman (1983) found that almost all mothers knew the basic 'growth=health' message and that more than 50 per cent were familiar with more specific messages regarding oral rehydration, Vitamin A, and others. In terms of these general messages, kaders have been successful health communicators. However, the weakness in their ability to adapt this information to the needs of individual mothers and children with specific problems has not been remedied. This continues to be an important challenge to the programme.

The technical performance of kaders on tasks has been assessed in various studies, with mixed results. Managing growth monitoring in the community can be difficult when mothers and crying children descend in large numbers on a few kaders. There is a tendency to focus on weighing and recording weights, rather than interpreting them and talking with mothers. The process of weighing and plotting requires some confidence with arithmetic and literacy, as well as systematically following a sequence of tasks to assure accuracy. BKKBN's (1986) study of kader programmes in East Java and Bali reported low levels of kader knowledge and technical proficiency. Allen and Goodwin (1988) carefully observed growth-monitoring activities, reporting that weighing and charting was done without significant error 60 per cent of the time—a pretty good record, and 75 per cent of the kaders were able to interpret the growth charts correctly. However, only 21 per cent of mothers received any feedback from the kaders on the growth of their children. This study commented that 'lack of communication remains the biggest obstacle to growth monitoring success'.

Unfortunately, we have no data yet as to whether the *Pos Yandu* approach will contribute significantly to improving these aspects of programme performance. Routine participation of health centre staff in community-based activities can have several benefits, including adding more person power to the sessions, ongoing supervision and guidance to kaders, and direct inputs to mothers and children.

Behaviour change

Identifying growth faltering, and informing and counselling mothers are expected to lead to changes in child care and feeding behaviours. These are the main mechanisms for programme impact.

The BKKBN (1986) study investigated numerous specific items of programme-provided information and related behaviour, exploring associations with attendance and weighing sessions. The results were mixed. There was high awareness of the significance of growth monitoring, but only moderate attendance at weighing sessions. Programme messages related to feeding of colostrum, frequency of child feeding, and an introduction of solid foods did not show much impact. Knowledge about the risks of diarrhoea and use of ORS was higher, with 36 per cent of mothers in East Java, and 45 per cent in Bali, reporting use of some kind of oral therapy in a previous epidsode. Immunization coverage was still fairly low (BCG under 50 per cent, DPT, measles and polio about 20–30 per cent), but both knowledge andpractice were significantly associated with attendance at weighing posts.

Fajans and Sudiman (1983) reported that many practices targeted by programme messages had been significantly modified in their small sample of successful programme villages. Similarly, Manoff International (1984) reported significant rates of adoption of specific changes in child feeding practices, with resulting improvements in child growth. This reflected one year's input of more intensive, carefully designed nutrition education and communication modules in a controlled study in five subdistricts. These results suggest that the potential for behaviour change and impact is there, although often not reached in routine implementation.

Impact on health and nutrition status

There is little basis in the information available for confident conclusions about programme impact. Only one study (Manoff

International 1984) provided a pre– and post–test design with control groups. This assessed behavioural and nutritional status changes in response to an intensive nutritional education/communication approach, and showed strong positive results. This suggests the feasibility of significant impact, but is not representative of the larger universe of kader programmes.

Fajans and Sudiman (1983) felt that, despite the high level of programme implementation and behavioural responses they found, there was 'no association between programme participation and nutritional status'. BKKBN *et al.* (1986) could also not establish any reliable links between programme coverage and health or nutrition improvements. They do report a positive relationship between weight-for-age of the younger children and attendance at weighing posts, but noted that weight-for-age measures were distorted by misreporting for ages.

THE COSTS AND FINANCING OF CHW ACTIVITIES

Despite the windfall from oil exports in the 1970s—sorely diminished in recent years—Indonesia remains a lower income country, still struggling to develop its health care system, and to reduce avoidable mortality and morbidity. Kader programmes have included significant public and private costs, in terms of both the resources of government used to support programmes and the contributions of communities and participants. How large are these costs? Is the money well spent? How much can be afforded? Some answers are available to these questions.

Programme costs: government and community

There are two major components to the cost of kader programmes in Indonesia: the financial resources put in by government and the uncompensated contributions of communities. Both of these components should be counted in estimating the total social cost of programmes.

In addition, the components are interesting in themselves. The cost to government represents the budgetary implications of supporting community-based programmes and should be compared with the total resources available as well as with the costs of alternative programmes and their relative efficiency and effectiveness. The uncompensated cost to communities is, in effect, their 'payment' for these services. Since in Indonesia's hierarchical society this is only partly voluntary (as discussed earlier), government support for kader programmes mandates, to some extent, community 'payment'. One might also ask how large is the size of this payment overall, as well as in comparison with the costs of other health services for which communities could pay?

Affordability

Sources of costa data on kader programmes include hypothetical costing models as well as empirical studies of programme costs in field settings. Results from some of these studies are summarized in Table 2.4. Frankenberg (1978) modelled both the government and community costs of generic *Pos Yandu*, based on field data from one district in West Java. She reported a total annual cost of about \$230–290 per *Pos Yandu* (roughly \$0.23–0.29 per capita, with an average *Pos Yandu* coverage area of 1000 population). Over 40 per cent of the cost was the communities' uncompensated contribution to the programme.

In 1986, UNICEF estimated the recurrent costs of village level activities, excluding contributions of villagers, as ranging from \$24–38 per *Pos Yandu*, with the number of posts per village ranging from two to eight. Investment costs were estimated to be \$87–143 per *Pos Yandu*. Assuming five-year amortization of investment costs and a population of 1000, this gives a total per capita cost of about \$0.06. Their estimate for the value of contributions from villagers was, however, much higher, ranging from \$112–152 per year per *Pos Yandu* in new villages (with community time contributions for initial training) to \$107 per year in old programme villages (UNICEF 1986).

In terms of field studies, a 1981 assessment of government costs in a kader-based pilot project, covering all villages in a single subdistrict, estimated annual per capita costs of \$0.61. Full coverage of villages with this resulted in a 40 per cent increase in subdistrict health expenditures in comparison with a similar control area without kader programmes (Berman 1985).

More recently, a detailed costing of government inputs to *Pos Yandu* development and maintenance in West Sumatra reported the average annual cost of maintaining a *Pos Yandu* at about \$100, not

Table 2.4 Cost and affordability of CHW programmes

Study/year	Field data/costing model	Total cost per year per Community post*	Estimated per capita cost†	Cost per output	Comparable clinic service cost/output
UNICEF-Jakarta 1986	Model	\$52–55 govt. \$107–152 community	\$0.06 govt. \$0.11 community	NA	NA
Frankenburg 1987	Model	\$229–289 old/new *Pos Yandu* includes govt. and community	\$0.23–0.29	NA	NA
Berman 1985	1981 Field data 1 subdistrict	NA	\$0.61 govt.*	\$0.19	\$0.46–0.51
Berman *et al.* 1988	1987 Field data 1 province	\$100–190 old/new *Pos Yandu* govt. only	\$0.20	\$0.50	\$0.44–0.78
Department of Health 1988	1988 Field data multiprovince	\$734 (about ⅓ from community)	\$0.73	NA	\$0.32–0.81‡

* Assume 5-year amortization of investment costs and annual recurrent costs.
† Assume average *Pos Yandu* population of 1000 if actual population figures not available.
‡ Estimate from national rural health service cost study in Berman *et al.* (1989).

including the communities unpaid contribution (Berman *et al.* unpublished data). The per capita cost was about $0.20 per annum for maintaining 100 per cent coverage in that province. This is equivalent to about 25 per cent of current government health spending on primary care services only.

A national study of *Pos Yandu* costs was completed in 1988 by the Department of Health *et al.* (1988). This study reported an average annual total cost per *Pos Yandu* of about $734, of which about one-third represented uncompensated community contributions. Assuming approximately 1000 people per *Pos Yandu*, this averages about $0.73 per capita per year—considerably more than has been shown by other studies. This may reflect differences in methodology. The study also found large variations in costs in different provinces.

The gist of these studies is that even a volunteer-based CHW programme requires a significant level of spending to achieve high coverage. The per capita costs are well within total government health spending of $2–3 per capita per year (Brotowasisto *et al.* 1988). The West Sumatra and West Java studies suggest that about 25–40 per cent of current government *primary health care* (PHC) *spending* is needed to meet the government's contribution. This is affordable given current levels of public sector health expenditure. Significant increases in resources for *Pos Yandu* are likely to be required to sustain this effort, although such inputs may be available from reallocations. The recent national study conducted by the government presents a more sobering picture. It reported much higher costs which, if accurate, would require large increases in resources to maintain.

Cost-efficiency

Comparisons of the costs of kader-provided services with clinic-based services suffer from the criticism that the two sources of care are not equivalent. Attendance at a community growth-monitoring session and receiving advice and supplies from a volunteer is not the same as a visit with a paramedical worker during the well-baby clinic at the health centre. While there is merit in this criticism, the comparison is still worth making—the two services are similar. The data show that the programme costs to the government of the kader contact are about 40 per cent of the cost of a clinic visit (Berman

1985). In the costing of *Pos Yandu* in West Sumatra, the difference was not as large. The total programme cost, including contributed community resources estimated to be equal to the government programme cost, would erase most, if not all, of these differences. However, when opportunity costs of the use of clinic-based services, such as users time and transport expenses, are considered, the community-based service may again be more cost-efficient.

These calculations suggest that, in terms of costs alone, there is likely to be a net benefit to community members of CHW services, even when community contributions are included. The provision of services in the community offsets the time and travel costs of users. This subsidy is likely to be especially significant to the more vulnerable lower income groups, which may explain why their participation in kader-based programmes has been proportionally greater.

While services provided through kader-based programmes have often been shown to be more cost-efficient than clinic-based services, their average costs may still be fairly high. The West Sumatra study reported costs per contact of \$0.50 compared with health centre per contact costs ranging from \$0.44 to \$0.78 for different types of services (Berman *et al.* 1988). Since *Pos Yandu* contacts occur monthly, the total annual cost per beneficiary of services is relatively high. This is related to the low number of beneficiaries seen each month and the fixed cost of regular visits by health centre staff.

Cost-effectiveness

While it is important to know the financial costs to government, communities, and beneficiaries in assessing the affordability and efficiency of CHW programmes, it is their effectiveness relative to cost that indicates whether they are an efficient strategy for public sector expenditures intended to improve health. While no studies have been done that explicitly assess the cost-effectiveness of kader programmes in comparison with alternative strategies in Indonesia, one can draw some conclusions from the data already cited.

An earlier paper by Berman assessed the cost-effectiveness of large-scale CHW programmes in six countries, including Indonesia (Berman *et al.* 1987). That paper characterized the programme as one of low cost and low effectiveness. It also noted, however, that routine PHC services were not necessarily much better in terms of effectiveness, although they were likely to be more costly. In such situations of low efficacy and productivity of public services, simple classifications of different strategies of service provision as more or less cost-effective are not very helpful. The main problem is how to improve both the effectiveness and efficiency of public services. Different approaches to this goal might include strengthening one mode of service provision while abandoning another, or integrating different components of the delivery system within a strategy of overall improvement.

Taken in isolation, services provided through Indonesia's CHWs continue to have lower average costs than other sources of care. CHWs' short training, limited skills, and high turnover result in likely low efficacy of the services they provide. In other words, on their own, CHWs are not a very cost-effective strategy for improving public health.

The more recent development of *Pos Yandu* may greatly improve the cost-effectiveness of CHW activities. It may have the added benefit of improving the cost-effectiveness of the health centres and sub-centres that make up the bulk of the public sector's PHC system. These facilities are now characterized by low utilization relative to capacity—meaning that average costs are high (Berman *et al*. 1989*b*).

The *Pos Yandu* strategy includes several components likely to increase cost-effectiveness. First, it may increase the clinical efficacy of services provided in the community, through the direct and regular attendance of qualified paramedical staff at village weighing sessions. Second, it requires that currently under-used clinic personnel spend more time in the villages, which will certainly increase the overall output of services. Third, it takes advantage of the community organization efforts of kaders to focus on times and places where those needing services will be present. And fourth, it gives priority to a package of basic services most likely to have significant public health impact.

Despite these positive developments, the data on *Pos Yandu* suggest that such effectiveness gains cannot be reached or sustained without significant increases in costs. Sufficient resources must be available to support the training, travel, logistics and supply implications of this massive health care extension effort. Successful *Pos Yandu* will probably increase the demand for curative care as well as for referral services. These will require improved staff and supplies. Cost-effective PHC is not necessarily cheap, and recent data indicate that Indonesia is spending considerably less than $1 per capita on rural primary care services (Berman *et al*. 1989*b*). This may not be sufficient to sustain successful *Pos Yandu* efforts and strengthen the capacity of clinic and hospital-based referral services.

It is difficult to assess whether other strategies might not offer better returns in terms of cost-effectiveness. One alternative would be to focus more on development of sub-centre facilities covering several villages with small teams of paramedical workers, avoiding the training, supervision, and supply requirements of large numbers of community-based health workers. The question may be moot at this time, given the high level of public commitment in Indonesia to *Pos Yandu* approach. It may be more important to focus on assuring the effectiveness of *Pos Yandu* and on improving the cost-effectiveness of the PHC system as a whole.

CONCLUSIONS

Major accomplishments and constraints

In little more than a decade, Indonesia has developed one of the world's most extensive programmes of community-based PHC. This programme is powered by voluntary action by communities, challenging the widely expressed doubts about the viability of volunteer CHWs. A vast majority of the country's rural and urban communities have access to volunteer health and nutrition workers who provide information to enable mothers and children to improve their health, along with a few simple health-enhancing technologies. Professional health workers are increasingly sent into the communities to work alongide these volunteers, increasing people's access to, and hence the coverage of, more sophisticated services.

As with any programme of this size and scope, there are both significant achievements and important problems. On the achievement side, communities, and especially mothers, are now widely familiar with basic concepts of the linkage between child feeding, growth, and health. Many mothers have learned how to measure and recognize important signs of impending health problems and have adopted methods for managing them in the community.

The involvement and contribution of communities to activities focusing on their own health improvement is palpable and impressive. Despite the effects of social and economic class distinctions, which are certainly important in communities, CHW activities often involve a spirit of mutual assistance and co-operation. Villagers devote resources to public health activities and provide an important link for the introduction of new services and programmes.

Indonesia's CHW efforts have signalled a strong emphasis on providing services where people live, as opposed to an exclusive emphasis on formal health facilities. Action to improve the health and nutrition of mothers and children is firmly established as a significant focus for government and community. The more recent development of *Pos Yandu* formalizes an active link between clinic-based personnel and the villages. It should improve the utilization and outreach of staff from health facilities, as well as strengthen the clinical efficacy of village-based services.

A number of serious constraints also characterize CHW efforts. From the inception of government-sponsored CHW schemes, it was decided to limit the role of kaders to primarily providing simple health information and to organizing villages for weighing and feeding sessions. These limitations persist today. Kaders themselves lack confidence in their roles and villagers often share this scepticism. Training of less than one week is clearly insufficient to provide much technical skill. Volunteer kaders receive little in the way of abilities, compensation, or supervision, offer few significant services to villagers, and frequently resign or reduce their efforts. The result is low coverage within villages and community activity limited to a narrow range of health-related actions whose efficacy is questionable. As community knowledge and expectations improve, this type of worker has little future.

The diffusion of community-based activities to many individual villages and hamlets places great demands on time and travel for clinic-based personnel. If attendance within villages is low, this time and travel commitment is much less worthwhile. Large numbers of CHWs also require a certain amount of support, such as supervision, retraining, and supplies, whatever their output. The relatively high average costs of specific *Pos Yandu* outputs, such as immunizations (Berman *et al.* unpublished data), reflect these factors. In addition, such poor performance reinforces the limitations of community-based services. Villagers may become understandably sceptical and uninterested, thus further reducing coverage.

High profile national efforts, such as the development of the *Pos Yandu* concept, can energize these activities for a while, but such momentum cannot be sustained for long purely on the basis of new ideas and priorities. Ultimately, the success of this, or for that matter any, configuration of PHC in Indonesia will depend on strengthening the efficacy and productivity of service resources. This will require much more support for things like kader training and retraining, supplies for community activities, travel and transport for supervision by clinic staff and attendance at community-based sessions. Community health efforts must also be supported by adequate services at referral facilities such as health centres. All of these requirements imply more resources for PHC.

Priorities for the future

What specific strategies should be considered for solidifying the accomplishments of CHW efforts to date, and for improving the efficiency and effectiveness of PHC into the future?

Community-based workers must have greater knowledge and skills than they now acquire. This may mean more substantive initial training, as well as regular opportunities for additional training. Increased supervision and contact with health personnel may also serve a training function. Improved kader skills might require more materials and supplies to be provided to CHWs, adding to the need for logistic support. More time for community health activities may also be needed. An important issue to be resolved is the extent to which these changes would be compatible with the type of part-time volunteer CHW now working in Indonesia.

Strengthening the quality and depth of community-based activities will also increase the work-load of health centres and sub-centres. The monthly visits of clinic staff to each *Pos Yandu* require a large commitment of personnel—over 50 per cent of total health centre staff time in some estimates. Currently, resources for travel and transport, staff incentives, and drugs and supplies are probably insufficient to sustain this level of effort. Administrative procedures are also a constraint. If an increasing demand for clinic-based services is also anticipated, new staff, vehicles, and other inputs will be needed.

Given the history of low productivity of health inputs in Indonesia, management factors must also be addressed, preferably as the first priority. Resources already available at the primary care level (and other levels) are poorly used (Berman and Sakai 1992). New investments should at least be accompanied by improvements in administration and evidence that new staff and other inputs can be adequately employed.

Pos Yandu may succeed in raising the effectiveness and efficiency of the whole PHC health care system—not only the community-based activities. In order to do that, however, more resources and better use of resources are needed. Indonesia's CHWs can be a great force for health development, or a missed opportunity—form without substance. The latter alternative, already too familiar to Indonesia's village population, is maintenance of the existing low productivity, low impact public health system, with kader activities gradually declining into disuse until the next campaign is announced.

3

The current situation of Village Health Worker programmes in China

XUEGUI KAN

INTRODUCTION

In the late 1950s the Chinese created and began to use 'barefoot doctors' in an attempt to extend the basic preventive, promotive, and curative health services to the under-served rural population. It was hoped to provide a bridge between the community and the professional health service, to mobilize community resources and thereby overcome the difficulties in government health resources, and ultimately, to achieve more improvement in the health status of the people at a cost that the country could afford. Today, an impressive improvement in the health status of the Chinese people has indeed been made, with life expectancy of nearly 70 years, and infant mortality about 35 per 1000 live births, despite fairly low per capita income. Although many factors could have contributed to this achievement (for example, improvements in nutrition, education, housing, sanitation, and other policies in the health sector, such as the use of traditional medicine and family planning), the use of village health workers (VHWs) can at least be considered as one of the contributing factors. (For the purposes of this chapter VHWs include only barefoot doctors and their successors—village doctors and health aides.)

The use of barefoot doctors has been seen as a Chinese model, and has inspired many countries to make substantial changes in their own health care delivery systems by launching a variety of VHW programmes towards the care of rural and urban poor populations (Rifkin 1980; Rohde 1983). At the time that these countries adapted the Chinese experience to their own, few had however made a thorough analysis of the particular political, socio-economic, and organizational basis on which barefoot doctors were introduced, and the underlying factors which could influence their success. Many problems have been raised since the national political and economic reforms of the last decade.

The 1970s and 1980s have seen significant political and socio-economic changes taking place in Chinese society, particularly in the rural areas. The unitary system of the collective co-operative economy in these areas has been replaced by many types of production responsibility system. Preliminary evidence suggests that these changes have been a great challenge to nearly all dimensions of the Chinese health system, especially to the financing of VHW programmes. What remains unchanged, however, is the 80 per cent of the rural population who are still under-served, and the fact that the country's health resources are still scarce. Having recognized these contradictory points, the Chinese health authorities have launched several policies attempting to maintain the valuable rural health forces.

This chapter will give a brief review of the historical development of VHW programmes in China, the socio-economic change of the country in the last decade, and its impact on VHW programmes. Several policies launched by the Chinese health authorities will be introduced and some comments will be given.

HISTORICAL BRIEFING ON THE DEVELOPMENT OF VHWS IN CHINA

Before the founding of the People's Republic, the health status of the Chinese people was extremely poor, with life expectancy of only 35 years, and infant mortality over 200 per 1000 live births. It was recognized by the new government that measures should be taken to provide basic care for people, especially those in rural areas, but the country could not afford hospital-based curative medicine by using government-paid medical workers. To deal with these very difficult situations, the central government formulated the national principles of health care in 1950, with four main emphases: providing health services to the people; putting prevention first; integrating traditional and western medical care, and launching health campaigns. Following these principles, continuous mass health campaigns were launched throughout the country, and multi-sectoral committees for health campaigns were established at different levels of administration. These health campaigns not only advanced public awareness of health issues through active participation, but also brought about widespread acceptance of communities' responsibility in the improvement of their own health.

At the same time, the government made available resources to build up the local public health system. The establishment of county health institutions (hospitals, epidemic prevention stations, and maternal and child health) was speeded up, and private medical practitioners were organized and integrated into joint clinics, usually located in townships.

With the development of health campaigns and the recognition of the fact that it was still difficult for many poor farmers to gain access to basic health care, interest concentrated on health services at village level. A co-operative medical service system commenced in 1955 and developed rapidly after the people's commune movement in 1958. This medical system was established on the basis of voluntary mutual aid and co-operation, by relying mainly on joint financial supports from the village collective welfare funds, villagers' personal contributions and on community-based insurance. The benefit entitlements offered by the scheme varied among brigades, but villagers were generally entitled to substantially reimbursable services and drugs at the brigade health stations and also at higher level health units. Because the system matched with the main ownership of collective economy in rural China at that time, the government gave very strong political support, so that it spread to the whole country by the late 1960s.

Barefoot doctors

Accompanying the co-operative medical system was the development of village part-time health workers, initially named *banongbanyi* and later called 'barefoot doctors'. By 1975, the number of barefoot doctors had reached 1.56 million and this constituted a major part of health manpower in rural China (Table 3.1).

Although all barefoot doctors did provide basic curative care, there was a strong emphasis on preventive and promotive activities. The detailed duties varied from area to area but, in general, they had the functions of (1) organizing local health campaigns; (2) carrying out disease prevention and maternal and child care; (3)

Table 3.1 Numbers of village health workers (VHWs) in China

Years	Village doctors	Health aides	Total
1970	—	—	1 218 266
1975	—	—	1 559 214
1980	—	—	1 463 406
1985	643 022	650 072	1 293 094
1987	723 799	554 700	1 278 499

* These village health workers used to be called 'Barefoot Doctors' and since 1981, when a new assessment started, this name has been replaced by the names 'Village Doctors' and 'Health Aides' (see text). (Source: adapted by the author from MOPH (1987).)

treating common diseases; (4) referring more complicated cases to higher level units; (5) health education and promotion; (6) guidance of family planning, (7) collecting and reporting health-related information (Zhou 1984).

The minimum three-month initial training usually took place in commune health centres, either with staff from local health centres and county health institutions, or with members of mobile medical teams, which were a very common practice in cities during the 1960s and 1970s. Continuing education was usually through regular visits of barefoot doctors to the commune health centres, and supervisory visits by health centre staff to brigade health stations. There were also some occasional refresher courses, according to needs.

Barefoot doctors were completely accountable to the villages which selected and supported them, and of which they were equal members. They were directly managed by brigade committees, and the role played by the staff of commune health centres was to provide technical supervision and guidance. No evident conflict between technical supervision and village accountability was reported, and the reason for this was perhaps the very strong political support for the programme. Under the commune system in the 1960s and 1970s, commune members were paid in the form of grain, as well as a certain amount of cash, according to the number of workpoints earned by each member. Barefoot doctors were usually remunerated in exactly the same way as other commune members, although in most cases their workpoints were counted slightly higher than the average. They were not allowed to charge commune members for services.

During this period, health care in most rural areas was totally funded by the communities themselves, with the exception of some simple equipment, supplies such as vaccines, family-planning devices and training subsidies, which were provided by local governments. This decentralized policy not only facilitated community commitment and involvement, but also ensured the job satisfaction of barefoot doctors.

SOCIO-ECONOMIC CHANGES IN RURAL CHINA DURING THE LAST DECADE AND THEIR IMPACT ON VHW PROGRAMMES

Following the decision to construct the 'Four Modernizations', a series of social and economic reforms have been undertaken during the last decade in rural China, and these have resulted in unprecedented changes.

The economic structure in rural areas has been changed from the unitary form of the collective co-operative economy to multiple forms of economy, that is, a combination of multiple forms of ownership. A variety of contract systems of work responsibilities have occurred; the family contract system in most cases, and the group contract system of various scales in others. Collective productive labour, in the form of the production brigade and team as a whole, has been replaced by individual labour, in the form of the family as a unit. The product distribution to a family will completely depend on the quality and quantity of the individual labour the farmer puts in (PBCCPEC 1987).

The job structure of rural labour, which has been stable for a long time, also changed after the reforms. More and more labourers stopped farming and moved to small rural enterprises (State Statistical Bureau 1987) and this brought about rapid development of the rural economy. The living standards and incomes of farmers rose rapidly (State Statistical Bureau 1988).

Meanwhile, the administrative and productive system of the commune, the production brigade and team, have been replaced by the township and village system.

These unprecedented political and socio-economic changes have been a great challenge to primary health care (PHC) and VHW programmes in China, and have produced new situations that these programmes have to face.

Expectations

Farmers' expectations of health care are continuously rising. A survey conducted in Shanghai county (Gao 1987) showed that some farmers were no longer satisfied with the simple health care in village health stations. Of the farmers surveyed, 18.6 per cent preferred to be cared for at county hospitals, and 13.4 per cent at township health centres. This situation confirmed a survey in Suzhou (Gong 1986), which showed that the number of out-patients treated at city or county hospitals had increased annually, while patients cared for at village health stations decreased rapidly. This report also suggested that pressures had increased from these farmers for better equipment, the latest medical technology, and better service quality and knowledge from the VHWs.

Partly because of these rising expectations, and partly because of the rising price of medical materials during the reform, the costs of the health services were increasing. At the same time, it was proving even more difficult to gather collective welfare funds, since the collective economy system had been abolished. As a result, the proportion of villages with a co-operative medical system significantly declined—from over 90 per cent in 1979 to less than 10 per cent in 1986 (Zhu 1988; Zhu *et al.* 1987).

Remuneration and attrition

The abolition of the co-operative medical system and the shortage of collective welfare funds have brought about great difficulties for the remuneration of VHWs. Unlike the situation before the reforms, when VHWs could obtain an equal, or even better remuneration than other farmers, now the work of VHWs could not be compensated reasonably, to accord with their time spent and their responsibilities. Some VHWs have had to rely on other channels to maintain their incomes, leading to a very high attrition rate. According to a report in 1984, 153 of the 522 VHWs in a suburban county of Beijing dropped out (Huaiyou Health Bureau 1986). Similar situations have also been reported from other areas of the country (Wu and Xiao 1988; Zhang 1986; Zhou 1986). Shong (1988) analysed the reasons for attrition for 37 VHWs who used to work at 31 village health stations in Xiaoshan County, Zhejiang, and later dropped out, and showed that 25 (68 per cent) went because of low remuneration.

Training and funding

Financial constraints for VHW programmes have also led to difficulties in VHWs' training. Training fees for VHWs used to be provided by production brigades in the form of workpoints, with a small subsidy from local governments. On-leave training usually did not influence the incomes of VHWs during training. After the reforms, however, VHWs themselves in some areas have had to pay a part of their training fees, because of the shortage of collective funds. Many VHWs are unwilling to spend a long time in training, when they do not get sufficient compensation. A report from Henan analysed constraint factors for VHWs' training and showed that answers from 44 per cent of the VHWs were 'no time', from 42 per cent were 'too expensive' and, more impressively, answers from 95 per cent of the village leaders were 'no collective funds to support' (Wang and Deng 1988).

Ideology and the role of VHWs

Perhaps the most important impact of the reforms on rural VHW programmes has been the ideological changes of village leaders concerning the role of VHW programmes. These changes were reflected in a survey conducted in Henan province which showed that 64 per cent of village leaders preferred individually run health stations (Shi 1986).

POLICIES LAUNCHED BY THE CHINESE HEALTH AUTHORITIES TO DEAL WITH THE PROBLEMS

These constraints became so critical that many people doubted the survival of VHWs in the newly changed society. On the other hand, the majority, both health authorities and lay people, have never changed their belief that China needs some kind of auxiliary health workers to provide basic health services to the large rural population, at a cost that both the community and the government can accept, and, that government-paid health workers cannot play

Table 3.2 Managerial forms of village health stations, China, 1987*

Managerial forms	Numbers	%
By village collectives	300 315	37.2
By VHWs jointly	82 966	10.3
By VHWs privately	363 285	45.0
Resident points by township health centres	29 141	3.6
Others	32 137	4.0
Total	807 844	100.1

* There were 721 327 villages in China in 1987 and 634 267 of them (87.9%) had village health stations. The total number of these health stations were 807 844 because some villages had more than one. (Source: adapted by the author from MOPH (1987).)

this role, because of both their small numbers and the inability of the government to pay them at the present time. Facing these contradictory points, the Chinese health authorities have launched several major policies in an attempt to tackle these problems and to maintain VHWs for PHC in rural areas.

Multiple managerial forms and financial patterns

The Ministry of Public Health (MOPH) has taken a decentralized policy to allow the autonomy of local governments in determining managerial and financial forms of VHW programmes, according to local socio-economic situations and the willingness of communities. As a result, multiple forms of management and financing have emerged. According to the statistics by MOPH (1987), the main forms of village health stations include: (1) those managed by village collectives, which own the station, decide how to raise funds and how to pay VHWs, and manage the station through village health committees or village committees; (2) those managed by VHWs jointly, which is the same situation as above except that the station is managed by VHWs jointly, where villages have more than one VHW, and payments are decided by both the village committee and the VHWs, usually under contract or norms, (3) those managed by VHWs privately, where individual VHWs run the station, raise funds, and get income through fee-for-service (Table 3.2).

Table 3.3 Percentage of different managerial forms of village health stations in selected provinces, China, 1985–86

Provinces	Percentage of different forms By village collectives	By VHWs jointly	By VHWs privately	Resident points by township health centres	Others	Total
Shanxi	84.3	2.9	11.4	1.4	0	100.0
Neimong	10.5	7.9	75.0	2.6	4.0	100.0
Jilin	68.0	4.0	28.0	0	0	100.0
Heilongjiang	88.5	6.6	4.9	0	0	100.0
Anhui	12.7	4.8	77.8	4.7	0	100.0
Guangdong	45.3	7.5	34.0	7.5	5.7	100.0
Yunnan	35.2	2.9	50.5	1.9	9.5	100.0
Sanxi	35.8	14.8	44.4	0	5.0	100.0
Hebei	51.6	3.4	43.9	1.1	0	100.0
Henan	24.2	3.4	68.7	1.5	2.2	100.0

Sources: DMA (1986); Fu *et al.* (1987); Shi (1986).

These different forms are not distributed evenly over the country and results from several surveys are illustrated in Table 3.3. The most significant change in financial patterns is that fee-for-service has become a very common practice. Village financing is decreasing in practice, and in places where it is still operating, other funding sources, such as drug sales, are used in conjunction. In most areas, local government usually allocate some funds to VHWs' training and subsidies, but the amount is very limited. Unfortunately, there are no surveys which analyse the detailed distribution of different financing sources.

Multiple sources and methods of VHW's remuneration

VHWs' remuneration could come from local government health funds, from village collective funds, from village enterprises and drug sales or from fee-for-service. A national sample survey (DMA 1986) showed that proportions of funds from different sources varied greatly among areas (Table 3.4). Methods of paying VHWs are also different. In some areas VHWs rely completely on fee-for-service and in others they may be paid in the form of salary. There

Table 3.4 Remuneration of VHWs in eight provinces, China, 1985

Provinces	No of VHWs surveyed	Percentages of renumeration from Local government	Village collective funds	Drug sales and service charges	Others	Total
Shanxi	135	7.6	63.5	28.6	0.7	100.0
Neimong	111	5.6	15.0	74.5	4.9	100.0
Jilin	55	9.9	42.3	34.7	13.1	100.0
Heilongjiang	139	11.7	48.9	16.4	23.0	100.0
Anhui	91	1.2	1.1	96.6	1.1	100.0
Guangdong	137	0.7	47.3	47.5	5.4	100.0
Yunnan	217	13.5	7.7	78.8	0	100.0
Sanxi	143	0.1	16.3	76.4	7.2	100.0

Source: DMA (1986).

are also some VHWs who get their payments from village health funds under contract or working norms, or by using a so-called 'floating allowance', whereby a portion is drawn from the fixed allowance of VHWs and is returned to them at the end of the year, in proportion to their service quality and quantity, as evaluated by township health centres (MOPH 1984 and 1985).

VHW's training and re-evaluation

The initial training of VHWs now usually takes place at county health training centres. The funds for training are mainly provided by local governments, with a variety of support from the community, depending upon local situations. A new assessment schedule for VHWs has been in operation since 1981. A certificate of 'village doctor' is offered to those who have passed formal examinations, or are qualified to have reached a level of health school graduates. For those who fail, the name 'health aides' is used.

Reinforcing the role of township health centres in the support and supervision of VHWs

Several ways have already been tried and some are still in the pilot stage. In order to strengthen local government support for PHC and co-ordination with village committees, the leadership of township health centres in some areas has been shifted from the county health bureau to the township government (Wu 1987). The prevention and PHC group within the health centre, which is the supervisory body for VHWs, has been strengthened by being given more autonomy and being allocated more staff and budgets (He 1987; Xiao *et al.* 1988). A contract scheme between the health centre bureau and local government has been established in some areas, in which the responsisibilities of the former in supporting PHC and the budgetary allocation by the latter are defined (MOPH 1985; Changshu Health Bureau 1986).

CRITICAL ISSUES FOR THE FUTURE DEVELOPMENT OF VHW PROGRAMMES IN CHINA

By the end of 1987, there were about 1.28 million VHWs working in 807 844 village health stations in 634 267 different villages (87.9 per cent of the total 721 327 villages in rural China). Of these VHWs, 60 per cent had been conferred certificates of village doctors, and the other 40 per cent were called health aides (Tables 3.1 and 3.2). There are other health personnel working at the village level, but their numbers are quite small compared to VHWs, and they are not multipurpose workers. For example, the only task for the part-time birth attendants is midwifery (Wu YM 1988; see Table 3.5).

It seems, therefore, that the total number of VHWs in the country has kept stable since 1985, and they are still the major part of health manpower at the village level in terms of their number and coverage. It is only in villages without VHWs (12.1 per cent of the total) that villagers have to seek services from other personnel. What is unclear but more important, however, is whether these workers are still working towards the goal of PHC. There are several critical issues for the future development of the VHW programme in this country, which should be considered further by the Chinese health authorities in their policy-making.

Functions of the VHWs

First, what are the main functions of VHWs? Are they multipurpose workers with emphasis on preventive and promotive activ-

Table 3.5 Categories of health personnel at the village level*

Categories	Number of health workers	%
Village Doctors	462	39.2
Health Aides	492	41.8
Private practitioners	47	3.9
Retired doctors	12	1.0
Doctors from township health centres†	14	1.2
Part-time birth attendants	120	10.2
Others	32	2.7

* Data from 1985 National Sample Survey of Rural Health Services, adapted by Wu Y M (1988).

† Doctors from the township health centre who live in the village and therefore can provide services in their spare time.

ities, based on the eight essential components of PHC defined by the Alma-Ata Declaration, or are they simply medical practitioners with most of their time spent in curative activities? Although there have been no follow-up studies on VHWs' activities within a defined area, preliminary evidence has suggested that time spent in preventive activities by the Chinese VHWs has been decreasing. A sample survey of 57 barefoot doctors in Shanghai County in 1980 (Gong and Chao 1982) showed that 12 per cent of their time was spent in preventive and promotive activities, but another survey made in 1984 suggested that this percentage was only 4 per cent (Young, quoted in Jacobson 1987). Another survey in Jilin (Zhang 1987) showed that the preventive services provided by VHWs in privately run village stations are much less than those provided by VHWs in collectively run stations. If this trend is still apparent, as it probably will be, then the only visible result of the national PHC plan could be damaged.

Financing the VHW programmes

Second, how do we assess the possible impact of the fee-for-service policy in financing VHW programmes on the goal of PHC? Although such a policy has to a certain extent lightened, the financial difficulty facing the village collectives and the government through cost recovery, it could be a great challenge to the realization of the goal of PHC. Vaughan and Walt (1983) have pointed out that if VHWs are allowed to charge fees, they will become more profit-oriented, private practitioners. They might, therefore, tend to select more curative than preventive and promotive services, because the latter are usually less profitable, and discourage the real health needs of villagers, particularly the poorest ones, which would lead to problems of inequity. If they overprescribe medicines, the burden of villagers themselves might increase and the overall cost of services might increase too, leading to low efficiency. Training and continuing education may also be weakened because of time considerations by VHWs, and this could also lead to low-quality services. The overall effect perhaps is a backward step from the co-operative scheme, in which more equitable services were provided through risk sharing (even though it was very limited), and VHWs were functioning more comprehensively towards the goal of PHC.

Strengthening support to VHWs

Third, how do we continue to strengthen community support? Obviously, the success of the barefoot doctor programme in China was largely dependent upon full political, managerial and financial support from the community, as well as technical support from the health sector. Bryant (quoted in Ofosu-Amaah 1983) argued that if the VHWs were functioning effectively, this was more likely due to failures in these relationships than in the activities of the VHWs themselves. Two recent case studies of CHW programmes in Colombia and Botswana by the Evaluation and Planning Centre, London School of Hygiene and Tropical Medicine, have again emphasized the importance of these supports to the success of a CHW programme (EPC *et al*. 1988; Walt *et al*. 1989).

Although the Chinese health authorities have continuously given their full support to these programmes, it is clear that community support has been weakened since the economic reforms. Without strong support from the community where VHWs work, the health sector's own support could have the danger of professionalism, loosening the links between VHWs and their communities and weakening their bridge functions. It seems that this issue has not yet been fully recognized in China, or careful consideration given to appropriate policies to remedy the situation.

All these three issues are critical to the realization of the national goal of PHC in China. There is an obvious need for both further study and policy reconsideration if current difficulties are to be overcome.

4

Community health workers in Nepal

CLAUDIA McCONNELL AND
MARY TAYLOR

INTRODUCTION

Community health worker (CHW) programmes have been implemented in a variety of ways, both prior to and following the 1978 Alma-Ata Declaration. In Nepal, the first training programme was initiated in 1979. Community Health Leaders were selected to improve the coverage of government health services, particularly in rural areas.

Following a series of reviews in the 1980s a new programme for training Community Health Volunteers was implemented in 1988. In contrast to past efforts, this programme focuses on the training of rural village women with the aim of addressing maternal and child health (MCH) problems. It is similar in design and content to many other programmes around the world.

Given the extended scope of the new programme it is important to examine the successes and failures of past attempts, so that lessons learnt can be applied to the training and support of what will amount to the largest work-force in Nepal's health care system. In this chapter we describe the way in which CHW programmes in Nepal have developed. We consider the problems that have been encountered, describe the way in which these have been tackled, and consider the way in which international health policies and donor priorities have shaped the development of these programmes.

BACKGROUND

Nepal is a small land-locked country situated between Tibet and India. The population of approximately 17 million is predominantly rural and widely scattered throughout the mountainous and rugged terrain. It is one of the poorest countries in the world (UN figures) and over 90 per cent of the population is dependent on agriculture (World Bank 1979).

The spectacular scenery and relatively untouched countryside that attracts thousands of tourists annually is also a formidable barrier to development. The urban population of the *terai* and the capital, Kathmandu, has access to piped water, basic sanitation, electricity, and motor transport. Elsewhere these amenities are rarely found and most communication and transport is by foot.

Political structure (See endnote, p.124)

The village *panchayat*, itself divided into nine wards, is the basic administrative and political unit. Approximately 30 *panchayats* are found in each of the 75 districts making up the 14 zones. Elections for representatives to the *jilla panchayat* (district assembly) are based on the *panchayats*. Since the referendum in 1981 there is universal franchise for election to the *Rastriya panchayat* (national assembly) as well as direct election for ward representatives. Each district sends one or two representatives (depending on population size) to the national assembly in the capital, and His Majesty the King makes direct appointments to this body. The government is represented in each district by officers from the different line ministries, whose activities are co-ordinated locally by the Local Development Officer and the Chief District Officer.

Agriculture and nutrition

The majority of the population is engaged in agriculture, producing a variety of staple crops (rice, maize, millet, potatoes) for home consumption. Pressure on available land is intense because of erosion and population increase, and even the relatively fertile southern plains are reaching saturation point, as hill farmers compete with Indian immigrants for space. The average farm size of less than one hectare conceals the grossly unequal distribution of land: recent statistics indicate that despite considerable attempts to intensify land redistribution, the wealthiest 10 per cent of the households produce over 46 per cent of the country's total income, while the poorest 20 per cent produce only 4.6 per cent of this total (HMG National Planning Commission 1987).

Small scale surveys have reported that between 50 and 70 per cent of households are not food-sufficient (Conlin and Falk 1979). For those with insufficient land to produce their annual food requirements, the opportunities for off-farm employment are limited—portering jobs in the dry season, agricultural labour, and seasonal migration to India. Food deficits are commonly met by selling off assets and accruing debts. The situation for many hill farmers is illustrated by the following extract:

> . . . Household members will always need to be prepared for stresses that could result from a poor harvest (due to rain failure or landslide) or from unexpected demands for expenditure (such as the payment for treatment received during illness or the expense of a funeral). They will also have to contend with diminishing yields from their land (because of loss of soil fertility) and the effects of inflation on the prices of food, kerosene and consumable goods. They will try to accumulate reserves of cash or to invest in assets that can easily be sold (such as livestock). They will try to diversify their production, taking up additional crops (such as vegetables and fruits) that can easily be marketed, yet do not reduce their capacity to produce staple foods. They will therefore be interested to find out more about opportunities for increasing production and/or income offered through development programmes. However, as they become involved in new initiatives, household members will need to invest more time in economically productive work. They will have less time available for child care and their children's health and nutritional status may well be compromised. (Nabarro *et al*. 1989)

The National Nutrition Status Survey carried out in 1975 found that 48 per cent of children under the age of six years were stunted, 3 per cent were wasted, and 4 per cent were both wasted and stunted (HMG Nepal 1975). No large, national surveys have been carried out since this time, but several smaller studies indicate that malnutrition rates among children and adults remain high, and that access to land, seasonal availability of food and prevalence of infections are important determining factors (Nabarro *et al*. 1987, 1988). A 1987 UNICEF/Nepal situation analysis of children indicates that decreases in infant mortality have not been accompanied by improvements in nutritional status (UNICEF 1987).

Vitamin and mineral deficiencies are significant problems. One baseline study found that 78 per cent of mothers were clinically anaemic (New Era 1986). Iodized oil injection programmes have been implemented for several years now, but an earlier survey found the mean national prevalence of goitre to be 58 per cent of the total population, with an estimated incidence of cretinism as high as 10 per cent in some areas (GCEP 1987). The prevalence of Vitamin A deficiency has also been reported to be moderately high in Nepal (Brilliant *et al*. 1985).

Health status and health services

The health problems in Nepal are typical of many developing countries, characterized by high infant, child, and maternal mortality and high crude birth and death rates. The majority of infant and child deaths result from the common infectious diseases including diarrhoea, pneumonia, immunizable diseases, malnutrition, and problems associated with prematurity and low birthweight.

Traditional faith-healers (*jhankris*) are still the primary and often only source of treatment for many Nepalis, particularly in rural areas. For those that can afford it, private practice is available, as is the profitable over-the-counter sale of drugs in most urban centres. The *Ayurvedic* system of health care is being institutionalized slowly, but is not as well developed, or used, as it is in India.

Since the 1970s the government has been committed to the integration of primary health care (PHC) services to ensure maximum coverage of the population. In 1975, the Integrated Community Health Services Development Project (ICHSDP)* was established to supervize the integration of all vertical health activities through the basic delivery unit of the health post. In addition to a variable number (depending on the level of integration achieved) of medical assistants, nurse-midwives and administrative staff, each health post supports and supervizes multi-purpose village health workers (VHWs), who are responsible for outreach work in the surrounding *panchayats*. Overall supervision of health service delivery in the district is the responsibility of the District Public Health Officer, based in the District Public Health Office (DPHO). Supervision and control of the district hospital is provided by the Medical Officer. The post of District Medical Officer (DMO) exists

* Formerly known as the Integrated Health Services, and the Community Health Integration Project. Its current name is used throughout the text.

in the government's long-term health plans, but this has yet to be sanctioned. The DMO is designated as head of the DPHO.

Following the Decentralization Act of 1982 there has been an effort to proceed with decentralization of planning functions to the district *panchayat*. This is a system-wide effort covering all sectors. As a separate process, and specific to the health sector, some management responsibilities that were previously the prerogative of the Ministry of Health have been decentralized to five regional health directorates. However, this new policy has yet to be made fully operational, and many of the staff posts necessary to ensure its viability have not been filled.

In practice, both in 1979 and the present day, the services available in rural areas remain extremely limited. Many hospitals and most health posts have no piped water, electricity, or facilities for surgery; constant shortages of drugs, staff, and equipment severely hamper the quality of service offered; morale is very low among staff who are actually in post; and the services themselves are generally underutilized. In most areas a committed health assistant with initiative, and access to a drug store to supplement his supplies, can achieve as much in offering curative care as can a doctor in a district hospital. The health service staff have little credibility with the population they serve, and little opportunity to improve their position when the allocation of budgets, drugs and equipment remains highly centralized.

The government and donors have renewed their commitment through strengthening the role of districts in programme implementation and the role of regions in providing support. District health teams are receiving training in budgeting, stock control, and staff management, and these initiatives are likely to enhance their ability to maximize the resources they have. However, there is little chance that health care will be accessible to the majority of the population within the next ten years, and the government recognizes the need to recruit ward-level volunteers as a means of ensuring that some preventive and curative services are made available at this level. It was this concept that resulted in Nepal's early attempts to involve 'the community' in programmes designed to improve access to health care (The Community Health Leader Programme).

THE COMMUNITY HEALTH LEADER PROGRAMME

The major criterion for the design of the pilot project (which was carried out jointly by the health department and the Britain Nepal Medical Trust) was that 'any new activity should complement, rather than compete with, the VHW programme already started, and . . . should be feasible on a large scale' (Chauls and Rajbhandari 1980). The first objective of the project was to train 3000 volunteers by 1985.

Village health workers

These workers are employed to provide the full range of integrated services at village (*panchayat*) level. As existing health posts become integrated, local (preferably), young (usually), males (nearly always) apply for posts at the DPHO and attend a six-week course at a regional training centre. They are paid a monthly salary by the district office to carry out a rigid house-visiting programme in their *panchayat* (3–5000 population). Their job description and tasks are similar to those in many countries: to carry out preventive and promotive activities and refer individuals to the health post. Although not given training in the use of drugs they often carry some to treat minor ailments. At the end of each month they spend three to four days at the health posts completing their extensive record forms for submission to the district health office. By 1978 some 1200 VHWs had been trained.

Much has been made of the inadequacies of the VHW programme and the oft-quoted descriptions of them as wall writers and 'the men that make the dogs bark' (Achard 1983). They are often physically unable to do more than mark the houses, given the extraordinary task they face in covering huge distances and altitudes. The whole concept of a 'village' worker seems to have been misguided in a country where very few nuclear villages and communities can be identified, either physically or culturally.

However, there were, and continue to be, other problems. This list is all too familiar. *Selection* criteria, which require that all government employees achieve the eighth grade in school, favour the children of the elite and male school-leavers. *Training* is inadequate in length and content, and practical field experience is minimal. *Morale* is often low, resulting from minimal job satisfaction and delays in payment of salaries and allowances. *Credibility* with the local population is poor, as the VHWs are unable to respond to the frequent demands for medicine, and are associated with the negative experience most villagers have of the local health post.

Assessments of the programme, while acknowledging that there were problems in selection, training and content of work, nevertheless focused on the logistic and administrative difficulties. Thus a new plan to overcome this problem was written in to the Sixth Five Year Health Plan such that:

> [The] Village will be the main focus for providing basic health services. As it will not be possible for the limited staff of the health post to perform this task alone, ward level volunteers will be utilised for this purpose. These volunteers will be trained by the Department of Health Services and through them the services of the integrated health post will be taken to the village level. (Nepal Planning Commission 1979)

Thus the Community Health Leader programme was conceived.

NGO involvement

As in many new programmes a non-governmental organization (NGO) was involved in part of the pilot project. Two HMG health posts (one in the Central Region and one in the Eastern hills, where the Britain Nepal Medical Trust had a health post visiting programme) were selected as initial sites. The Britain Nepal Medical Trust (BNMT), a non-governmental organization, has been working in Nepal for twenty years, primarily in tuberculosis control and community health. Since BNMT staff had been working on VHW strengthening activities they were in a good position to help add the new dimension of the ward level volunteer.

The staff working with VHWs had reached the conclusion that they were unable to visit houses frequently enough to have any effect, and that some new way of working had to be evolved (Groman and McConnell 1978). Earlier attempts to rework VHW schedules in the context of ongoing work at health posts had not been successful. Finally, in the Mamling Health Post area, VHWs were granted permission to bring villagers together for meetings instead of visiting every house.

These meetings presented the first opportunity (in most areas) for people to sit together and discuss health and related issues. Interested individuals would accompany the VHWs on their rounds and contribute to subsequent meetings. Gradually, the possibility of sharing the work-load with such a volunteer was discussed among the VHWs themselves. They liked the idea of selecting an individual who was known to them within each ward, or discrete subgroup within a ward, and sharing the work of teaching and motivating villagers. Some VHWs had quite serious communication problems with people from different ethnic groups who frequently, particularly the women, had a poor grasp of Nepali: a volunteer from each ethnic group could go some way to resolving this. Similarly, the VHWs liked the idea of the volunteer being responsible to 'his/her ward', and felt that this would have a beneficial influence on selection and motivation.

Government plans and policy

In 1978, the National Planning Commission issued a preliminary policy document (prior to publication of the Sixth Five Year Plan), which stated that one important target was to provide a health worker in each ward by the end of 1985. A high-level task force consisting of the chiefs of all the vertical projects (Malaria, Family Planning and MCH, Leprosy, and Tuberculosis) was convened, with external assistance from a USAID-funded advisory group.

The experience that ICHSDP had gained in implementing a small pilot project (training ward-level volunteers) led the task force to recommend that the job of such volunteers should be more substantial than merely providing support to health post and VHW activities. Lengthy discussions about the job description and recruitment procedures followed, and were complicated by the need for each of the vertical programmes to ensure that their programme area was at least as well represented as any other. This struggle for power and control over a new cadre of worker (who, we must not forget, was supposed to be a community worker) was most clearly manifested in the writing, field testing, and revision of the Community Health Leader (CHL) training manual. Conceived for use by barely literate people, the final labour produced a 200-page document which received minimal field trials.

There were two other issues which emerged as crucial, both for determining the way the programme was implemented, and for the influence they had on subsequent changes and the evolution of the most recent volunteer training programme. These are payment and selection of women.

Involvement of the clients of the CHL's services in their selection, supervision and remuneration was considered to be a vital element in their potential 'success'—and a vital difference between them and the VHWs, who were government employees. While acknowledging that CHLs were unlikely to work for nothing (although this was tacitly assumed at the start of the programme), the planners and NGOs involved felt that some form of remuneration from clients was needed—both to make the programme financially viable and as a demonstration of 'commitment'. It was therefore assumed in project documents that each Ward Health Committee (WHC), established prior to selection, should devise its own mechanism for supporting the CHL. This could be in the form of fees for service, fixed charges per household, or payment in kind or labour.

The second issue that was hotly debated, particularly within the project implemented by BNMT, was whether His Majesty's Government (HMG) or, in this case, the Ministry of Health (MOH) should actively determine that women volunteers were selected by stating this in the project guide-lines. Women were likely to be more acceptable to clients, but were unlikely to be selected through traditional mechanisms at ward level. In the end the issue was side-stepped by saying that each ward should be entrusted with responsibility for its own selection, but would be 'advised' to consider the advantages of choosing female volunteers.

The pilot project

In 1980 the project was implemented in Naubise (Dhading District) and Mamling (Sankhuwasabha District) health posts and CHLs from each ward attended the health posts for the initial 12 days of training. Prior to this an orientation programme for District Public Health Office (DPHO) and health post staff was organized by national-level staff.

Although the pilot project carried the weight of HMG involvement, there was little genuine enthusiasm for the programme. Much of the commitment and pressure to continue came from the donors and involved NGOs, who were anxious to ensure that Nepal was seen to have a real expression of PHC services as outlined in the

Alma-Ata Declaration. Over the next five years, ICHSDP trained over 4500 CHLs in 16 districts. This coverage was achieved by recruiting US Peace Corps volunteers to initiate and supervise the training programme.

The original CHL concept was now being implemented in two rather different ways. The Ministry of Health, with Peace Corps, were anxious to increase 'coverage' quickly by meeting targets of the number of volunteers to be trained nationally. Meanwhile, the NGOs were exploring the process in more detail by focusing on the effectiveness of the volunteers in a few villages and wards. In the most general terms, the MOH and some donors were concerned with quantity, while NGOs were concerned largely with the quality of the programme in a small area.

Reviews of the CHL programme

Several reviews of the national CHL programme were undertaken. These reviews were carried out in response to donor's needs to document progress as well as to plan for future resource allocation. In 1982, a conference was held which identified the following problems: lack of community participation; ineffectiveness of VHWs in their supervisory role; lack of motivation in the absence of incentives: and minimal involvement of women. Conference participants proposed modifications of the implementation strategy, in particular that Ward Health Committees should be encouraged to consider selection of female CHLs. The programme continued essentially unchanged (HMG Nepal 1982).

A comprehensive review was also carried out in 1987 with USAID technical assistance that was 'to assess the present status of the CHV Programme effort and the desirability and direction of continued USAID support' (Taylor 1988). (From the time of this review the term CHL was dropped in favour of CHV.) The findings of the review were positive in so far as 63 per cent of CHLs were still active in their communities, both health post staff and villagers felt that they had contributed to some health activities, and their presence had stimulated the communities to be interested in HMG-provided health services. The problems identified were very similar to those mentioned in the 1982 review, and revolved around implementation issues. Specifically, the CHLs and WHCs failed to replenish initial supplies and were thus unable to meet their clients' demands for curative services; orientation of the community was not carried out well and WHCs were therefore inactive; 90 per cent of CHLs were men and were not reaching village women, especially for MCH and family planning services; and CHL morale was low since they were neither recognized, supported, nor resupplied. Management problems in central and regional level MOH structures left districts unsupported, often without budgets and materials. In addition, the MOH at that time did not have a clear, ongoing and meaningful policy commitment to the support and integration of CHLs in the health care system.

In summary, the CHL programme was developed and initiated with considerable support and pressure from the major donors and NGOs. It was seen from the outset as a means of improving outreach of the PHC services without incurring much additional government expenditure. The lack of orientation and involvement of potential clients, and of clear policy commitments, led to the subsequent decrease of interest and support from those who had been instrumental in initiating the programme, resulting in its slow death. In areas where intensive and innovative support had been sustained, there is some evidence that clients want, and are prepared to support, the services provided.

THE COMMUNITY HEALTH VOLUNTEER PROGRAMME

In 1988 there were major changes in the organization and leadership in the MOH. District and health post level services were restructured into a more integrated, decentralized system. Policies and programmes were also influenced by the Basic Minimum Needs Strategy which was being adopted at the time. Both placed emphasis on the CHV as the community agent and 'cornerstone of integrated health service delivery' (HMG National Planning Commission 1987). Several influential individuals became involved and the MOH developed a comprehensive implementation strategy for a 'new' programme for women, by women. It was announced that CHVs would be deployed to cover the entire country by the year 2000.

The most radical departure from previous policy was that all CHVs would be women over 25 years, married, and willing to volunteer in their wards. Female CHLs would be selected and retrained in the new programme. Male CHLs would be encouraged to continue voluntary or paid work, but would no longer be the focus of MOH activity. Strong political support for the new programme was expressed through the Royal Family, the Prime Minister, and the Minister of Health.

Strategy statements outlined a new programme beginning with the creation of one 'mother's group' per ward. The concept of a mother's group was based on pilot groups that were formed for the purpose of supporting family planning and MCH work. The mother's group would select the CHV, and then meet monthly with her to discuss, learn about, and try to solve some of the health problems in their own villages. By activating and using these support groups it should be possible to resolve some of the earlier programme's problems with community orientation and ongoing support. It should also enhance the ability of the CHV to tackle health problems that are largely affected by improving access to information and changes in behaviour.

The MOH also officially chose the Nepal Women's Organization (NWO) as a partner in orienting communities, selecting CHVs, and providing ongoing support to them. The NWO is a political organization (one of six organizations directly aligned with the present system of government) with the purpose of providing a distinct and formal voice for the women of Nepal. While the NWO did not exist in all areas at the start of this programme it was the largest organization representing women in Nepal. The MOH hoped to build upon the organization, and use its networks to organize mothers groups and CHVs. District, zonal, and central levels of both organizations would meet regularly together to review CHV programme implementation.

Other problems that had been identified in the CHL programme were considered and addressed. Remuneration was partially resolved by offering a 100 NRs per month ($4.00) honorarium through the government. Resupply of drugs was addressed by proposing that the initial supply of materials should be sold to the CHVs, who in turn would be encouraged to charge their clients for their use, essentially creating a revolving fund.

Implementation

In 1988 HMG established a target of providing 12 days training to over 14 000 CHVs. To achieve this several activities were planned:

orientation of central, regional, and district level personnel; development and production of training curricula and materials appropriate for non-literate village women; training of district health post staff to be trainers; formation of mothers' groups in each ward, and selection of CHVs. By the end of the year supervision and support systems were also to be in place.

First year progress

Over 10 000 mothers' groups were formed, and training was provided to nearly all CHV candidates selected. A non-literate training manual was developed and well-received by trainers and trainees. Most of the district and health post staff in one-third of Nepal's districts have received some training as trainers of volunteers. Initial post-training analysis of a sample of CHVs showed that their level of knowledge and skills, related to diarrhoeal disease control and childhood immunization, were good (Taylor *et al.* 1989).

The timing of implementing the 1988 organizational changes in service delivery in the districts had a significant effect on the CHV programme. As with any major organizational change, decision-making about personnel placements and reorientation to new roles took precedence over many programme activities. This was especially true for VHWs. As these decisions were worked out and finalized it was difficult to define, let alone implement, the day-to-day management and supervisory support required by the new cadre of worker called CHVs.

In practice, guide-lines were given and plans implemented with the expectation that the programme would enjoy considerable resource and political support for the short term. It was intended to produce results quickly on a large scale, without full consideration of long-term resource needs. Thus tremendous effort was put into providing training, postponing supervision and support strategies until later.

Some issues arose that differed from earlier experience with CHLs. The relationship between the MOH and NWO was new, and the role of the NWO largely unspecified. Misunderstanding over the criteria for CHV selection, and the struggle for supervisory power ensued.

Management and logistical problems associated with training village women were sometimes significant. Training sessions were often interrupted and shortened to accommodate domestic responsibilities. There were not enough female trainers to effectively communicate family planning and MCH topics in a culturally appropriate manner. Simplifying the knowledge and skills that CHVs were supposed to have was difficult for health post staff, and not enough emphasis was put on the use of practical exercises to enable non-literate CHVs to cary out all of their tasks.

The programme also had to contend with the usual MOH management problems, including the late release of budget, delays in printing, and lack of staff. Pre-conditions for release of funds that were originally set to ensure a link between programme implementation and improved management systems did not have the desired effect.

Early reviews

The MOH and donor-provided technical advisors are currently reviewing the performance of CHVs during the second year of programme activity. Some anecdotal and early impressions have been noted through visits to some districts. Feedback from VHWs and other health post staff has been positive, and echoes the feelings expressed by staff in the CHL pilot project areas.

Active CHVs are functioning as referral agents for some kinds of services. Health post staff and coverage data indicate increased attendance at immunization camps, where CHVs have notified mothers and children ahead of time. More oral rehydration packets have been distributed from health posts and CHVs, compared to equivalent months in past years. Health post staff see the CHV as someone who they can call on to improve the use of services they provide, especially those services that have clearly defined targets provided by the central levels of the MOH. Particularly active health post staff make use of CHVs as go-betweens for reaching village women, and they attend mother's group meetings to do their own teaching about 'priority' services (Taylor 1989).

Problems have been reported with the resupply system, whereby CHVs sell bandages and simple drugs to their clients. This has introduced an element of distrust among villagers, who perceive that the CHVs are making a profit from the arrangement. The CHVs also do not sense that they 'own' the supplies when they are forced to purchase them with part of their training allowances.

Some have tried to remedy this by collecting several rupees from each household in their ward to pay them back for the initial outlay.

Acceptance of the CHVs in their wards has varied. In general, where political factions or highly politically active communities (including the NWO) existed prior to the CHV programme, selection and support problems have been encountered. Because of the pressure to ensure rapid implementation last year, a blind eye was turned towards most of these problems, and now some CHVs are not able to represent or teach effectively in their wards. In places where factions did not exist, or where there was a history of an active CHL programme, it has been easier for CHVs to begin working with mother's groups.

Perhaps most importantly, some women now feel that they have a crucial role in understanding and doing something about health problems that affect their children, regardless of whether they are literate and educated or not. They are also clear about their expectations. The 100 Rs per month honorarium is a major reason they (and in many cases their husbands) have agreed to function as a CHV. They are concerned that they may never receive this payment, or that it will not continue for very long. They feel they need more money to do things, such as provide tea during mother's group meetings or to travel around their wards.

It is not yet clear what CHVs as a group will be doing after the first year of activities. At the start, any new programme benefits from its newness, enthusiasm, high expectations, willingness to commit time, energy, and resources. Women have been specifically selected to carry out tasks that they did not already realize they could do. They are being paid, albeit a small amount, to do this. This might give them a sense of empowerment, or importance, that encourages them to continue without support or solutions to problems in the first few months.

It is also not clear what flexibility and problem-solving ability the MOH will be able to bring to bear on the implementation of the programme. There have already been changes in its project status reflected by very slow release of honoraria funds. During the past several months influential advocates for CHVs have been transferred to other ministries, giving staff fewer opportunities to make things run smoothly. Traditionally, the MOH has allocated resources and developed expertise in training, but much still needs to be done to develop and maintain the support and supervision systems that are necessary to any ongoing programme (Walt 1988).

ANALYSIS

The problems that were identified by informal and formal reviews of the CHL programmes can be grouped under four main issues: (1) involvement of women; (2) incentives and supplies; (3) management and supervision; and (4) community participation and policy commitment. In this section we examine the extent to which these problems have been addressed or resolved in the new programme, and the factors that have affected the ability of programme planners to build on past experience.

Services by women for women

The CHV programme has made some progress by clearly stating that women are selected and trained to provide services in their wards. Traditional, cultural, and political structures have a major influence on the role of women in Nepal. Women rarely seek or are granted positions of authority, and are seldom involved in decisions affecting community action. Women do not traditionally seek counsel from men regarding treatment for their infants and young children either, except when these men are traditional healers.

This problem was recognized by planners of the original CHL programme, but they were unable to overcome it despite repeated attempts at guiding both predominantly male health post staff and village leaders, except in one district where it was compulsory that all CHLs would be women. Learning from this experience, the new programme attempts to circumvent the traditional male dominated political structure by working through the NWO.

This decision has also allowed the MOH to take advantage of existing networks of women, and to tap their human resources to improve orientation and selection. But, it has also introduced problems that should have been anticipated at an earlier stage of planning. First, selecting the NWO had political implications at all levels, especially in rural areas. As with any existing organizations, especially those aligned to the political system, there are groups of women who belong and those who do not. In some areas the organization of women was viewed with suspicion, and in many cases NWO officers were often chosen by virtue of being related to the traditional male political leaders. As a result of these conflicts CHVs were not always selected as intended.

The inappropriate selection of CHVs will affect the success of the programme, especially where selected women are not married, or really willing to volunteer, or able to work with all groups in a ward. Programme managers, who have little record of being able to influence decisions, are now faced with trying to ensure that *appropriate* women are selected as far as possible, to ensure that more resources are allocated to orienting and communicating with NWO groups, and to ensure more effective co-ordination between the bureaucracies of the MOH and the NWO.

Incentives and supplies

After ten years of discussion on the subject of payment of incentives to CHVs, the MOH has decided to make direct payments of honoraria. While set at the low level of 100 NRs per month per individual, on a national level the recurrent costs are considerable: over 1.5 million dollars, or 7 per cent, of the national health budget (HMG 1988). If CHVs function effectively, it is possible that this is a worthwhile expenditure. However, in the current economic climate in Nepal, it is likely that other ministries and politicians will need persuading that $1.6 million per year spent on supporting non-literate village women in their work is a good use of limited resources.

Even at this time these funds come primarily from the MOH regular budget, since nearly all the donors have declined to pay recurrent costs for personnel. There is some indication that the delay in payments is partly a result of questioning by other ministries. In the original programme design, the community is expected to find ways of providing these funds once they are convinced of the CHVs' importance. However, the MOH does not specify how the new programme is going to stimulate such fundamental community ownership of activities identified by central-level planners. The MOH has provided a short-term answer for incentives, but has gone no further than with CHLs to work out long-term arrangements.

A related problem that plagues the entire health care system in

Nepal is resupply of drugs and first aid materials. The CHL review found that there was conflict between volunteers and clients over whether these materials were freely distributed or sold. This undermined the entire relationship between the two—and limited the credibility and effectiveness of the volunteer. The CHV programme introduced two changes to this scheme. CHVs were to purchase initial stocks rather than receiving them free, and health posts were to maintain resupply stocks with the money collected. This was to be communicated to district and *panchayat* leaders.

Medical supplies are always in short supply in the government sector. The private sector does not extend into all rural areas, nor is it always affordable. Health post drug supplies often last for only three to four months a year. It is unrealistic to expect the CHV revolving fund to solve the problems of resupply in this environment. District staff are likely to apply the management skills they have to stocking the health posts first, and it is possible that clients would prefer this also.

We see two areas of uncertainty in the new programme, and little obvious long-lasting change from the strategies used in the old programme. The MOH has stated that, over time, clients will be persuaded by the beneficial work of the CHVs to find ways to raise the funds for incentives and supplies themselves. While stated as a plan at the central level, no significant work has been done with either districts, health posts, or communities to devise feasible plans for phasing this support in. Past experience of the WHCs and health post committees has shown that, in most areas, clients were not willing to take responsibility for financial support of their CHLs. Although the government is now exploring mechanisms for cost recovery by charging user fees in selected health posts, the prevailing opinion of health care workers and clients is that the government will continue to provide free services, and CHVs are perceived as being part of the government system.

If such support is not forthcoming, the risk of losing the motivation of CHVs to work, in the absence of payment and supplies, is very high. The MOH may be faced with finding a solution to this problem with very little time to test alternative strategies. The lack of consultation at village level has resulted in predictable problems arising after the programme has been implemented.

Management and supervision

Traditionally, management skills have not been stressed in the training of health care workers. The levels of infrastructure, communications, and transportation systems in developing countries also make managing supplies, personnel, budget, and activities difficult. The CHV programme is being implemented in the management context of the MOH. This context has been well described in other management reviews, and much assistance is aimed at improving it.

Programme budgets are nearly always released one to two trimesters late. This means that all activities must be planned for the last half of the year, or be undertaken on the promise of funds to come. Since the funds available are not always sufficient for all activities, especially *per diem* costs and supplies, funding for activities already undertaken cannot be assumed. This has introduced distrust of the system, lowered morale, and made workers unwilling to take risks with their time. This affects the CHV programme to the extent that NWO, or ward members, are unlikely to undertake activities on the promise of funds that are controlled by government employees. In the first year, regions and districts manipulated resources to make CHVs a priority activity, and tried not to let late release effect implementation schedules. This was possible in a policy climate that made CHVs an important national priority, but may not be sustainable.

The MOH has a stated policy of decentralization of budgeting and planning. DPHOs and district *panchayats* are supposed to plan for, budget, and receive funds within ceilings, according to their own local priorities. In practice this system does not yet operate. Plans and budgets are prepared by districts, but most programme direction, activities, and budgets are still determined at central level. This tension is likely to continue as decentralization involves the shifting of power. As with decision-making and personnel, the timing of the decentralization of health system management is lagging behind what the CHV programme needs. Flexible local solutions to problems cannot be implemented by staff who feel constrained by guide-lines prepared at central level.

The personnel system of the MOH has undergone drastic change as workers were restructured out of vertical programmes into one integrated system. Many health posts are understaffed, especially with Assistant Nurse Midwives who are virtually the only female workers at this level. VHWs exist in number, but are not necessarily trained or stationed equitably throughout rural areas. CHV programme norms require many staff for training, supervision and reporting. The desire to meet training targets has often overridden the acknowledged need for sufficient staff to carry out activities well. This is especially true of activities such as supervision, the results of which are much harder to monitor than counting numbers of workers trained. Lack of well-trained staff, in the right place, and at the right time, continues to be a significant constraint for the CHV programme.

Management and supervision problems remain unchanged for CHVs and CHLs, with the possible exception of the size of the CHV work-force and the fact that they are all women. While the reorganization and decentralization of the MOH should contribute to more effective support of CHVs, there has not been enough time for the system to equilibrate and allow decisions to be made on the basis of greater local control and better placed staff. In an uncertain environment, with limited staff resources available to them, CHV programme planners have made decisions for the short term. These have favoured rigid programme guide-lines, emphasis on training, and postponement of support systems development. It should be noted, however, that the management problems have not really worsened, even though the CHV programme is far bigger (in sheer numbers) than the CHL programme. This is an accomplishment for the first year, although it may make supervision issues more difficult when they are finally confronted.

There are special questions that did not concern CHLs, but that should be asked about supervision for CHVs. The new CHVs are all women who will be supervised primarily by men, who are most probably not related and whose relationship will be dictated by tradition. Is it possible to forge a new relationship of mutual respect and teaching that will be necessary for CHVs to be successful? Will it be possible for males and females to interact and discuss MCH and family planning subjects? Past experience has shown that, with a few exceptions, this line of communication is not open. Is a new *panchayat* level of female worker needed? What referral systems can realistically be developed when health posts do not generally have female staff?

Community participation

It should, by now, be clear that both the programmes described are similar in design and orientation. Their purpose is to improve access to government health services through deployment of voluntary workers, whose financial support will be provided by the clients. The planning, design, and implementation of these programmes is carried out at central level, with little opportunity for flexibility. Thus, orientation activities are commonly described in terms of 'explaining to people what the CHV programme is', and 'ensuring that the community understands the level of support they should provide'. In this climate it is unlikely to have, and unrealistic to expect, committed participation in a programme which is viewed by the majority of its clients as an extension of the health services.

The CHL review stressed that time was an important factor in achieving adequate orientation, and recommended that orientation activities begin the year before any training. This was to allow sufficient time for staff to visit and carry out substantive discussions, formally and informally. In the implementation strategy for the CHV programme, ward-level orientation is not separated out as a discrete activity. Much of it is subsumed in the formation of mothers' groups and the CHV selection process. NWO Primary Committee members and VHWs are supposed to 'orient communities' while they are making lists of mothers and children under five years old. Health posts are to invite a village *panchayat* leader to all NWO primary care orientation meetings. While information was provided in a booklet that was used to orient regional and district level staff, no instruction or suggestions specifically tailored for village level were provided.

During the first year of CHV implementation, the need to meet government targets quickly caused the first several steps to be condensed into a one-month time period. Resulting problems with CHV selection were one indication of the gaps in the process. The CHVs have not been working long enough to assess the levels of support they will receive, but the shortage of time, and the lack of guidance and importance placed on this activity repeats the mistakes of the CHL programme. It is not clear whether it can be remedied through closer work with mothers' groups.

In essence, the MOH is struggling with the need to develop community participation and ownership of a programme that was designed by planners at central level. The MOH has stated it wants communities to find ways to support CHV honoraria and drug supply systems, although it does not allow comment or input from clients on CHV roles and tasks. While NGOs have shown some success on a small scale with an innovative development process, there are not many examples where it has succeeded through government on a national scale. The MOH in particular has not shown a capacity to allow flexibility in programme implementation. With both the geographical and political diversity in Nepal, it is unlikely that one 'programme' will succeed everywhere.

CONCLUSIONS

The Nepali government has made a clearly stated commitment to the new CHV programme. Policies have been formulated and recognized in the Basic Minimum Needs Strategy. The programme is well-meaning and, at this stage, supported both politically and financially. Why then are CHV programme planners implementing a programme that does not take into account many of the lessons learned about CHLs?

There is still a fundamental disjunction between the political imperative to implement a programme that will meet the requirements of the Basic Minimum Needs initiative and satisfy donors, and the major structural and administrative constraints that exist in the country. This disjunction leads inevitably to a repetition of strategies that work in the short term—ensuring that volunteers are trained and in place—but are not sustainable.

In this particular case of moving from CHLs and CHVs, the climate of organizational and personnel change in the MOH has also made it difficult for programme planners to propose solutions for any but the short term. One thing all CHV programmes with active community support require is time to develop appropriate strategies and relationships. The overall improvements in the CHL strategy, as seen in the CHV programme, may be the involvement of women. It is not yet clear whether this will open doors to mothers' changing behaviour, or demanding and using essential health services. It would seem from other national examples that issues of incentives, management and supervision, and community participation must first be resolved, or at least improved over time. The risk in the current CHV programme is that without these improvements, this time it will be women who fail.

Programme planners have designed a programme that tries to meet the needs of all the groups concerned. The Ministry of Health wants to improve coverage of the integrated health services. The major donors want Nepal to adopt the PHC strategy as outlined by WHO. The NGOs are keen to encourage 'community involvement' in health care. On paper at least, the programme is supposed to address 'community needs' for more autonomy and local control over resources. The original problem—availability of basic health care, especially to mothers and children—remains.

ENDNOTE

During the first few months of 1990 the *panchayat* government of Nepal was dissolved and an interim government was appointed until elections in May 1991. Despite changes in the political and administrative structures in the country, the issues addressed in this chapter concerning the management and sustainability of community health worker programmes remains substantially unchanged. The recent National Health Policy of His Majesty's Government of Nepal (published in English in October 1991) makes only passing reference to the role of women volunteers at ward level.

5

Community health work: India's experience

P. B. DESAI

INTRODUCTION

The purpose of this contribution is to reflect on the steps taken in India in the direction of universalizing access to primary health care (PHC) through a large cadre of what are called community health workers (CHWs). The creation of this cadre was initiated by the first ever non-Congress government, that of the Janata Party, on 2 October 1977 (the birthday of M. K. Gandhi, the 'Father of the Nation'). On that day, the government introduced their Rural Health Scheme, which was projected as a measure designed to place 'people's health in people's own hands'.

That government did not last long enough! The Congress was returned to power in 1980, retained the scheme, but made it a part of their Minimum Needs Programme, mounted to alleviate rural poverty. After about a decade of their rule, the Congress recently surrendered power to the National Front, dominated by the Janata Dal.

In ideology, the Congress (1947–77, 1980–89), the Janata Party (1977–80), and the Janata Dal (1989–) do not differ much; they all invoked Gandhiji's widsom and Nehru's charisma, and remained vacillating around the centre of the political spectrum. However, in their governance, the Congress leaned more towards Nehru than towards Gandhi, while the Janata Party pretended, and the Janata Dal now pretends, to be more Gandhian than any of the other parties. There was, therefore, no difficulty for the Congress in 1980 to retain the innovation of the CHW cadre that the Janata Party had introduced. Likewise, the new National Front government will in all probability carry forward the Rural Health Scheme.

What is not quite clear is whether they will let the scheme run as it has so far, or modify it to suit the prevailing circumstances. There are indications that the new regime wishes to pay more attention to social aspects of development, which, in their view, were neglected in the past, and also to shift the emphasis in planning to rural India. There is an expectation, therefore, that a rather sharp departure from the past is in the offing within the health sector, which will, in all likelihood, involve a deeper reconsideration of the CHW programme as well.

It is therefore opportune to reflect on the working of the Rural Health Scheme, and consider how community health work may be conducted more efficiently and effectively in future. Such an exercise is attempted here, with a view to demonstrating that the approach to PHC remains to be worked out, and there is little that the experience of the last twelve years has to contribute to this matter. Issues involved in the democratic dispensation of PHC in the current context will shape the future course of the country's pursuit of the Alma-Ata Declaration's goal of 'Health for All by 2000 AD'.

The discussion is divided into two parts: the first describes and comments on the performance of the CHW programme, and the second speculates on an alternative approach to 'Health for All' in the not too distant future.

THE RURAL HEALTH SCHEME: 1977–89

The timing of the Scheme is rather significant. The first thing to be noted is the compulsion for a new party in power to do something in this particular field, in order to sustain credibility in the eyes of the common people. In the preceding 30 years of their rule, the Congress had expanded national health services, including their rural component in a manner that had bypassed the rural masses. It had allowed the rural health system to be completely undermined by the non-medical, non-health programme of family-planning propagation it had internalized.

The latter programme had remained in a sort of drift for many years since its inception in the early 1950s. During the 1975–77 span of 'internal emergency' it was greatly intensified, with all the force at the command of an administration aiming to vasectomize rural males on a large scale, especially in the northern states. This caused massive political discontent against the Congress rule. The new Janata Party took advantage of this discontent and held out an election promise to free family planning from coercion or compulsion of any short, and to ensure people's undiluted access to health services in the rural areas.

Secondly, by that time knowledgeable circles in India, and in most of the developing world, had become thoroughly disenchanted with implanted allopathic medicine, despite its rapid technological progress. They deplored the neglect of indigenous systems of medicine, as well as the utter indifference to preventive, promotive, and rehabilitative aspects of health care involved in the proliferation of allopathic medical care. Indian planners and policy-makers had pronounced that the expansion of the medical services, in both the public and and private sector, was divorced from social, economic, and ecological realities pertaining within the country; that they were in no way related to the associated fields of nutrition, water supply, dietary requirements and habits, food preservation practices, and so on: and that they were largely confined to servicing the fads and fancies of the affluent classes in urban areas (Draft Sixth Five Year Plan 1979).

Outside the government, a high powered Study Group sponsored jointly by the Indian Council of Medical Research and the Indian Council of Social Science Research was actively debating an alternative model for the National Health System. They, too, denounced the existing health services, not merely as ineffective and unsuited to the needs of the country, but also as positively counter-productive to progress in matters of health. They advocated that 'the existing exotic, top-down, elite-oriented, urban-biased, centralized and bureaucratic system which over-emphasizes curative aspects, large urban hospitals, doctors and drugs should be replaced by (an) alternative model of health serivces . . .' (ICMR-ICSSR 1981).

This intellectual climate supported the political search for an alternative to the defamed family-planning scheme, and this materialized in the form of the Rural Health Scheme.

The National Health System

The National Health System that was then called upon to subsume the new implant of the Rural Health Scheme had had its own history of proliferation since Centralized Planning was introduced in 1951. The system had three principal components, which operated independently of each other. The first comprised a series of vertical programmes launched centrally to deal with major communicable diseases that took a heavy toll of life, such as smallpox, malaria, filaria, cholera, tuberculosis, leprosy, goitre, trachoma, and blindness. Each of these campaigns had its own specialists, leading a national corps of trained unipurpose field workers. By the time the CHW programme came in, the campaign against smallpox had been wound up, but its army of vaccinators had been retained to be accommodated somehow in the second component of the health services. Attempts were also well on the way to intergrate the personnel from these vertical programmes with those in the general health services. Unipurpose workers were being given reorientation training aimed at bringing them all together to form a unified cadre of multi-purpose workers (MPWs), who would then undertake the necessary field-work within the framework of the general health services.

The second component of the National Health System was the rural health services, which included family planning, to be delivered at the doorsteps of couples in the reproductive span of life. The process of creating the necessary physical infrastructure picked up during the Second Plan period, when the decision was taken to build Primary Health Centres in rural areas all over the country. Subsequently, it was decided to extend the outreach of these Primary Health Centres through the creation of a ring of Sub-Centres around them. This rural health and family-planning infrastructure comprised, on the eve of the Janata Party Government's Rural Health Scheme, 5430 Primary Health Centres, 38 594 Sub-Centres, 126 rural hospitals, 258 subsidiary health units, and 124 mobile units. They operated to provide some sort of health cover to a rural population of around 500 million. This infrastructure admittedly had yawning gaps in the provision of buildings, equipment, and vehicles. It was grossly deficient in different categories of qualified medical and paramedical staff, and the logistics of delivering these rudimentary services were out of gear for most parts of the country most of the time.

The health care that this system attempted to deliver remained virtually confined to clinical work; the system had no notion of preventive health care, except immunization of individuals carried out on a selective basis and on a modest scale. The work that the system was now required to undertake was family-planning propagation, with the emphasis on vasectomy, which was pursued with increasing vigour till it assumed unbearable proportions during the emergency. There followed a backlash, and the discredited programme could be circumvented only by redesignating it as a family welfare programme, involving a sort of integration of family planning with maternal and child health care. Under this new name, there was in effect a switch-over from vasectomy to tubectomy, which could be performed with great ease by the use of laparoscopes.

Where the infrastructure was reasonably adequate, there were several official community level medical and health workers within the jurisdiction of the Primary Health Centres, themselves provided at the rate of one for every 100 000 people. Apart from physicians and surgeons at the top of the hierarchy, there were health assistants, male and female multipurpose workers, nurses, lady health visitors, and midwives. At each of the Sub-Centres within the Primary Health Centre area there was an auxillary nurse midwife (ANM), a male MPW, and several trained or untrained traditional birth attendants (called DAIs) for a rural population ranging from 5000 to 10 000. Even so, the outreach of the rural health services was limited, confined in nature to clinical work and plagued with patron–client relations. What was of continued concern to these field personnel was the official expectation that they should concentrate on bringing family-planning cases to the Sub-Centres and Primary Health Centres, so that targets fixed for sterilization and IUD insertions could be attained. Indeed, this work often resulted in the loss of credibility of these workers in the eyes of the rural people they were supposed to serve.

The third component of the National Health System was medical education and training. Impressive progress had been made in the expansion of the medical education system that the colonial rulers had established. Medical colleges producing graduates in allopathic medicine increased from a mere 30 in 1951 to 109 in 1978, and their aggregate annual output of graduate physician/surgeons had increased during the same period from around 960 to over 14 000. Apart from this, several all-India institutions for postgraduate studies and advanced research, like the All India Institute of Medical Sciences, Delhi, were established, leading to a rapid expansion of facilities for clinical specialization and sophisticated research. Facilities for the training of auxillary and paramedical personnel had also been greatly expanded. This enlarging quantum of medical expertise, knowledge, and skills represented, however, only an aggregation of technologically upgraded medical care, and was clearly unsuited to the conditions prevailing in the vastness of rural India. Educational advance was, in fact, marginal in respect of the more important preventive and promotive aspects of health care. The educational system had, for example, remained impervious to subjects like public health, epidemiology, community health, and social medicine.

Introduction of Community Health Workers

Under the circumstances, the Rural Health Scheme came in to operationalize a new link between the village communities, on the one hand, and the National Health System, particularly its second component of Primary Health Centres and Sub-Centres, on the other. The link had to be operated through the Sub-Centre, which was the outermost, or peripheral, organ of the system, with three community workers, the male and female MPWs, and a traditional birth attendant helping the female MPW in MCH work. However, they were all perceived by the simple rural folk as agents of the all-powerful central government, and were to be feared rather than befriended. The fear was real, for the community level workers were observed to be emphasizing constantly the urgency of sterilizing fertile couples.

The solution that the Scheme worked out was admirably simple. It merely resurrected a 40-year-old prescription of the National Planning Committee (NPC), to the effect that there should be a health worker in every village who, by example and persuasion, might with missionary zeal spread in his own village 'the gospel of healthy living, communal and personal, and thus take the other villagers a step away from their age long prejudices and superstitions on the road to better living. He will not appear to villagers as a strange imposition of a strange system, but their own kith and kin who desires to help them'. This prescription is contained in the 1939 resolution of the NPC on the subject of public health. It was subsequently published in the Report of the Sub-Committee on Health (NPC 1948).

Strictly in line with this resolution of the NPC, the Rural Health

Scheme mandated that there should be in each village, or rural population of around one thousand, a CHW, whose job it would be to assist the people in getting their health problems resolved through the peripheral grass-root level organs of the National Health System.

The Rural Health Scheme envisaged that the village community would select from among its own members a person with modest education to function as a CHW. It was expected that the CHW would spare sufficient time from his regular vocation to provide, after receiving training for the purpose, adequate PHC to the entire population of his village, and educate them in matters of prevention and promotion. Specification of the duties of the CHW included treatment of minor ailments; giving first aid in emergencies; identification of cases of malaria, tuberculosis, leprosy, and other communicable diseases; rendering help to paramedics in their work related to communicable diseases, immunization, family planning and MCH, nutrition and mental health; arousing interest among the members of the community in environmental sanitation and personal hygiene, and actively promoting health education among the rural people. In principle, CHWs were expected to play a meaningful role in all the varied aspects of health care, in addition to facilitating the people's access to medical care. On the curative side, their role was strictly limited to administering first aid and treating minor ailments, an area usually not attended to in the villages. Beyond this, they were expected to refer all cases of illness to Primary Health Centres, Rural Dispensaries, or District Hospitals.

Newcomers into the health field were not to function as a part of the rural health services. They belonged to, and represented, a village community, who not only selected them for the job but were also supposed to regularly oversee their performance. They had, however, to depend on the Primary Health Centre of their area for logistic support, remuneration, professional advice, and technical guidance. The Scheme had specified that CHWs would receive, at the Centre, training for a period of three months in the new health functions they were required to perform for their community. During this period they were given a reasonable stipend of Rs 200 per month for their maintenance. After the training, they were given a token honorarium of Rs 50 per month, and furthermore, were to receive replenishments of the supplies they were required to carry in their kit while on duty (worth Rs 50 per month). During the training period, they received a manual of information and instruction on their varied functions, which they were expected to follow strictly, consulting it as and when needed in the course of their duties. The kit was given to them at the end of their training: it contained simple medicines and accessories, including dressing materials, allopathic drugs, and popular indigenous (*Ayurvedic*) medicines for common ailments.

The Scheme was introduced in October 1977 in the Primary Health Centres of all the 28 districts, where the reorientation of the unipurpose workers from the different vertical programmes had been completed, transforming them into MPWs. It was also introduced in one of the Primary Health Centres from each of the other districts where this transformation of unipurpose into multi-purpose workers had not been taken up. Altogether, 741 Primary Health Centres were involved and the total number of CHWs selected for training was around 8000.

Expansion and modifications

From this small beginning the programme of endowing a rural population of around 1000 with a trained CHW proliferated rapidly to envelope most of the country. During this period the norms of population coverage by different health institutions were changed, with a view to enlarging their clientele. As of today, provision exists for one Community Health Centre for a population of 100 000 on the average, and this is meant to serve as a referral institution for four Primary Health Centres; one Primary Health Centre should exist for every 30 000 people in the plains, and for every 20 000 in hilly, tribal, and backward areas; one trained CHW is provided for each village, or a rural population of 1000; and there should be at least one trained indigenous birth attendant for each village.

The total number of CHWs progressively increased in the course of the following decade to reach an impressive figure of 394 397 towards the end of 1987. This included 1420 health workers for the four States of Jammu and Kashmir, Kerala, Tamil Nadu, and Arunachal Pradesh, all of which had adopted alternative schemes to improve the outreach and performance of their rural health services. Under the Constitution, health is a State and not a Union (or Federal) subject, and so the States can exercise their right to operate an alternative to a centrally sponsored scheme. This occurs despite the attempt to achieve uniformity by the Central Council for Health, which is presided over by the Union Minister for Health and Family Welfare.

The course of the expansion of this cadre of CHWs has not been smooth. The centrally hatched scheme took a long time to reach the grass-roots. Various high level pronouncements about the scheme created quite a confusion on the part of the peripheral personnel of the health services, the CHWs and the rural communities. There was no clarity about the roles that these parties had to perform under the scheme. Communities could play a very limited role in the selection of CHWs, who were not clear about their status, and health personnel did not like the intended extension and activation of their functions. The CHWs assumed that they were 'Workers' attached to an important government agency; that their training enabled them to assume the role of a 'general practitioner', though less qualified than a medical graduate; and that they must receive the same amount throughout their career as they had received while under training. In fact, they could not distinguish between salary, a stipend, and an honorarium. Soon enough there sprang up CHW unions and associations to fight for their status and remuneration.

Meanwhile, the Central Government was also having second thoughts about its commitment under the Scheme. Towards the end of 1979, the National Development Council decided that the cost of the Scheme should be equally shared by the States and the Centre, and that the CHW should be renamed as a community health volunteer (CHV).

The response of the States to the decision on financial arrangements was entirely disappointing and most discontinued the Scheme. The reconsideration of the Scheme was not taken up in the following year, as the political situation changed adversely for the Janata Party. It attracted attention only in the middle of 1981, when the Congress government had established its full control at the Centre and in most of the States. As a result, in August 1981, a notification was issued to announce the revised centrally sponsored and funded scheme under which the CHV was renamed the Health Guide.

Apart from the change in the designation of the CHW, the new scheme was not fundamentally different; the only innovation it made was the provision for the villages to form their own health committees to monitor, guide, and supervise the work of the Health

Guides (HGs). Subjects specified for review by the Village Health Committee (VHC), comprising members with little knowledge of public health and no knowledge of medical care, were: (1) prevalence and control of communicable diseases, especially malaria, tuberculosis, and leprosy; (2) family planning; (3) maternal care and child health; (4) health education; (5) purification of sources of water supply; (6) seasonal illness and ailments; (7) environmental sanitation; (8) prevention of blindness.

This specification may well appear to be unrealistic, but the Scheme could not do less, as its defined objective was to secure community participation and prepare a cadre of volunteers, socially inclined and capable of being trained to provide PHC and health education to the community. If they were unfit or unable to take up this task on account of their limited knowledge and education, the Primary Health Centre and Sub-Centre medical and paramedical workers could do it on their behalf, and educate them in the process. The Scheme specifically ordained that 'as such the HG should be shown the same courtesy and high consideration as are due from public servants to any leader of the community. No doubt the health funtionaries would possess better technical knowledge and skills but these are to be used in guiding the HGs and VHCs in tackling the health problems of the community and not to assign the governmental funtionaries a higher status'. (Joint Secretary 1981).

Evaluation and criticisms

The CHW (CHV or HG) programme has been evaluated from time to time, both by official and non-official agencies. In response to the findings of these evaluation exercises, attempts have been made to ensure a better selection procedure for CHWs; to induct more females than males as CHWs; to prevent CHWs from assuming a greater role in medical care than specified; to improve co-ordination of their work with the work of grass-roots-level health service functionaries including ANMs, MPWs, Health Assistants, and Lady Health Visitors; and to invoke the interest of the rural people in matters of health.

No tangible success would appear to have been achieved by these attempts. For the most part, CHWs continue to treat minor ailments, participate in family-planning and immunization campaigns, and assist MPWs in their drives against communicable diseases. There is little evidence that the health situation has meaningfully improved on account of the performance of CHWs, except in stray pockets where high-cost specialized projects have been taken up by voluntary organizations. These pockets are too few to make any impression on the national health scene, and, in fact, any improvement in the national scene goes to the credit of alternative rural health programmes conducted by States like Kerala and Tamil Nadu.

The Scheme has been criticized on almost all counts, from the selection procedure, vitiated by the indifference of village communities and the inaction of Village Health Committees, to the quackery practised by the Health Guides. In general, rural folk are happy that they have an access to someone in matters of distress, but they would like them to be much more capable and influential, so that they can redress their complaints. However, the most damaging, but tactitly accepted, criticism is that CHWs have taken little interest in preventive, promotive, and rehabilitative health care.

It was anticipated that they would be a link between the village community and the health services. This has happened to some extent in the treatment of minor ailments, but CHWs have also operated to recruit family-planning cases. The link remains virtually inoperative in so far as progress towards the Alma-Ata version of PHC is concerned, because the community has not shed its age-old dependence on the official machinery, and is neither integrated nor united to undertake any exercise of self-reliance. In addition, the personnel of the national health services, even at their peripheral rural outlets, have not shed their bureaucratic and professional ways, and hibernate there as if in expectation of getting out at the first opportunity.

As a noted epidemiologist has remarked:

> the CHW Scheme was originally introduced for health promotion with better community participation and involvement, but now it is administered under the family planning programme and its sole purpose is to bring 'cases'. Added to this retrograde step, the health workers, male and female, have started using Health Guides as their substitute workers, instead of providing guidance and support to these persons who do not belong to the health services. Both MPW and CHW Schemes have been allowed to distort, degenerate and disintegrate because of administrative failures. They need to be scrapped in their present form. (Deodhar 1986)

Despite claims of its success reported by a series of evaluations conducted by agencies and institutions fully dependent on the government for their funding, it is clear that the working of the Rural Health Scheme has remained disappointing. To prop up the image of the CHW (HG) as a social leader by the fiat of a Central Circular has been of little use. HGs cannot become social leaders just by the government's saying so; success is assured only when established social leaders accept to operate as HGs. The fault does not lie with the mechanics of their selection, or with their application and commitment; it lies with the operative relations which have developed between the rural health services and the beneficiary rural people.

The services are incapable of tackling the larger tasks of the prevention of diseases and the promotion of health, while communities, hibernating in a state of disintegration wrought by colonial rule and left untouched (or perhaps aggravated) by government in the subsequent years of independence, have been incompetent to select their own health workers or to guide, supervise and monitor their work. As a result, the chosen CHWs used their new position to subserve the narrow rural power-base, and to patronize the poverty-sticken rural masses. In this they did not go beyond treatment of minor ailments, promoting family-planning acceptance, and facilitating immunization of those who came forward. The Village Health Committees remained ineffective in providing any guidance, and were oblivious of the possibility that CHWs can help the people to prevent illness, to promote health and obtain information, education, and training. They, too, saw them as the last link that extended the outreach of rural health services.

The health establishment had, to begin with, discounted the utility of the Scheme, but when they found that both the politics and the people desired the location of HGs within rural communities, they used their bureaucratic ingenuity to co-opt them as the most peripheral workers in the system. Since the communities were, for the most part, incapable of exercising any control over the HGs, the Primary Health Centres used their dependence on them for guidance, supplies and honorarium to render them pliant workers, who could save the health staff at the ground level a lot of the bother of dealing directly with the people.

Both when the scheme was launched and now, the factors inhibiting its success far outweigh whatever prerequisites may exist for its reasonable performance. The usefulness of having a CHW may not, even so, be questioned; what is at issue is the resurrection of the economically and socially shattered community organization, so that it can use a CHW to help itself to improve the health of its members.

AN ALTERNATIVE APPROACH TO HEALTH FOR ALL IN RURAL INDIA

These reflections on the performance of the proliferating cadres of CHWs, established under the Central Government's Rural Health Scheme of 1977, yield a rather disquieting conclusion that the work of the CHWs has made little difference to the course of development in the field of rural health. Their addition to the array of professional and paraprofessional employees, manning the national rural health infrastructure, now comprising over 1500 Community Health Centres, 12 000 Primary Health Centres and 55 000 Sub-Centres, has not resulted in overcoming the health services' clinical and family-planning biases, or the extension of their substantive scope and physical outreach, or in any improvement in their operational logistics. CHWs can claim no credit for the modest progress in national health reflected by trends in macro-level indices; the most that can be said of them is that they might have helped somewhat to reduce the perennial underutilization of clinical services, so long a feature of the health services in India.

At the ground-, or the grass-roots level, the health situation has, in any case, remained as grim as ever in most parts of the country. This means that the load of community work needed to make an impression on the grimness of the situation remains as large and as pervasive as ever. It is imperative, therefore, that we mount a serious search for an alternative strategy for the attainment of Health for All in rural areas as early as possible.

Though we are disappointed with the performance of the CHWs, we do admit that no alternative strategy can afford to ignore the crucial role that such a community-oriented worker must play in this adventure of attaining Health for All. Obviously, the notion that a CHW is necessary for upgrading rural health services was born out of the realization that the implanted professionalized, bureaucratized, and technology-oriented health services have failed in their principal task of improving rural health. That notion attracted a large measure of credibility when it was propounded at high policy-making levels; it even raised expectations that a sharp departure from the official approach to health would follow, to ensure the success of the CHW scheme. This did not happen. The introduction of the CHWs was not accompanied by any departure from the proliferation and working of the pre-existing health infrastructure and delivery systems, or by any change in ethos and ethics of the vested interests determined to preserve the *status quo*.

All aspects of the introduction and working of the CHWs have, accordingly, suffered neglect from the official establishment, and apathy from the communities they have tried to serve. The establishment transformed the CHWs into a peripheral, subservient link with the rural folk, who, though happy to have them in their midst, remained indifferent to their role as spokesmen before the health services in matters of medical cure, and as leaders in matters of preventive and promotive health care. In the circumstances, the CHWs formed a hanging bridge between the health services and the community. They were forced to work for the lower-level health personnel, particularly the MPWs, within the community, and yet shied away from the community, whose leading lights expected them to fight their own crusade against the sources of ill health inherent in the community and its environs. Unable to satisfy these expectations of community leadership, the CHWs became mere underdogs, tied at the lower end of the hierarchy of medical and paramedical professionals of the rural health services.

Impact of colonial rule on social organization and health care systems

One of the reasons for this unhelpful attitude of the rural folk towards the work of the CHWs could be their failure to recall their more distant colonial past, when the self-sufficiency of a self-reliant village community also embraced matters relating to medical care and public health. Even though its economic base was under communal ownership, that community represented a highly inequitous social structure, resting on a hereditarily determined stable social statification (the caste system). What is notable about this social organization is that, despite inequities, it ensured that in normal times the minimum basic needs of even its lowest stratum were satisfied.

Among these needs, health and medical care were given their due importance. The community had among its members a hereditary practitioner of the indigenous *Ayurvedic* medicine, who, as if by a religious injunction, served, without any discrimination whatsoever, all members of the community. In addition, there were several other part-time or full-time health workers, including an osteopath, a bone-setter, a nature-cure specialist, a yoga specialist, a midwife, and also a veterinarian. Together, they formed a team of CHWs whose services were available to the members of the community around the clock.

They were not paid by individual beneficiaries for the services they rendered: they received their due share in this respect from communal production, according to the *jajmani* system. Medical and health services constituted a communally remunerated social service, available equally to all members of the community, and not a scarce marketable commodity subject to profiteering, as it now is.

Admittedly, recalling pre-colonial village self-sufficiency is not helpful in the present context and is best left alone. Yet the impact of colonial rule on the traditional basis of social security needs to be clearly understood, for that impact has not been mitigated but accentuated, as far as large tracts of rural India are concerned. This is evident both in the viability of village communities, and in the deprivation experienced by rural masses in the matter of health care. The shattering of village communities' viability has left most of rural India in ruins, characterized through and through by abject poverty, deprivation, and injustice. Villages are there as they ever were, but the integrated communities capable of regulating the economic and social intercourse of their members, which they once represented, have vanished.

Today, a village typically comprises a large number of interest groups, or factions, based on caste, occupation, income, or political affiliation, pitched against each other for command over the shrunken resources within its jurisdiction. The invasion of market competition into rural India has eliminated all forms of traditional co-operation; this has shattered the fabric of rural social organization and thereby rendered it incapable of serving any of its purposes. It is this stark reality that generates scepticism about the capabilities of village communities to utilize the services of CHWs.

What CHWs could do was to facilitate the access of rural people to the health services provided by the government; that in doing so they accepted subservience to the paramedics of the services has been noted earlier. It must be emphasized here that public provision of allopathic medical care in rural areas has almost completely undermined the practice of a variety of time-tested indigenous systems, which represented a combination of curative, preventive, and promotive health care. It is well known that the allopathic system was brought by the colonial rulers to serve their army and civilian establishments. Up until Independence it was confined mainly to cities, cantonments, and larger towns; it selectively penetrated into the rural areas to the extent that Christian missionaries took up medical welfare as a part of their proselytization of the rural folk. After Independence, the penetration of allopathy into the countryside was achieved by the wide spread of the official rural health delivery system. Along with this, there was a matching expansion in the production of allopathic skills and expertise, a part of which, unable to compete in the urban market, entered rural areas to man these services. This rapidly undermined the traditional systems, for the simple reason that it was difficult for the rural people to cast off the spell that the quick-cure allopathic medicine had exercised on their unwary minds.

So, at a time when the mechanization of medical care is creating uneasiness in the western mind, whose product it was, it is finding a ready custom among the rich in the cities, towns, and villages of India. The mass of poor in rural and urban areas are deprived of traditional medicine; they aspire to allopathic cures, but simply cannot afford them, even when they are made available as a part of public services. The CHWs have made access to the public provision of allopathic cure for the rural poor a wee bit easier, but they have concentrated on peddling among the people the contraceptives (sterilizations and IUDs) provided by the same services.

Voluntary, non-governmental health programmes

Disintegrated and derelict village communities, and the inadequate and often counter-productive performance of the rural health services are the two principal elements against which we are left to speculate on the positive role that CHWs may play in lifting the standards of rural health. In doing so, we may cast a brief look at the accumulating experience of a large number of contemporary projects mounted by private charitable, philanthropic, and humanitarian concerns outside the government, in what is called the voluntary or non-governmental sector.

Human misery, caused by high levels of mortality and pervasive morbidity, evokes widespread concern and constitutes perhaps the oldest field attracting the benevolence of the rich, the well-to-do and the enlightened in society. From among the many forms that this voluntary action against ill health takes, we are not concerned with the most modern and the most sophisticated medical institutions, the five-star hospitals, created by the charity of the rich, or the *nouveau riche*. Most of them seek to combine medical care with medical research and training in order to benefit from tax exemptions available for the promotion of the general welfare of society. In any case, most of these five-star medical establishments are located in urban, especially metropolitan, areas and they have no place for any useful role that a CHW can play.

Our concern here is with programmes that seek to involve the community in the work of upgrading the standards of health of their members, and make use of voluntary workers drawn from their membership for that purpose. Apart from the penetration of Christian missionaries for dispensing allopathic philanthropy, there are in the vastness of India's human geography, innumerable institutions, organizations and groups who are engaged in the provision of medical and health care to the rural poor; often they combine this health work with social and economic welfare or development. Their motivations may differ, but almost all of them seek to activate rural communities to take upon themselves the task of improving their own lot. Invariably, they profess to be in search of models of health care that can be universalized in the developing world. It would be almost impossible to provide an overview of this vast ongoing experimentation in the establishment of health care facilities in rural areas. From among numerous such experiments that have been reported in the enlarging literature on health, two examples can be cited which seem to have made purposeful use of voluntary workers drawn from the communities covered by their respective projects. They can be said to constitute, by their differing approaches, the two ends of the range of health and medical services, extending from rudimentary community level health care to the most sophisticated medical services provided by a system, with a college-hospital as the apex of its referral hierarchy (Ford Foundation 1987).

The first of the two examples represents an extension of the activities by the Christian Medical College and Hospital (CHC), Vellore Tamil Nadu, into the field of PHC in one of the rural blocks in its vicinity. By any account, this is one of India's premier medical institutions, the excellence of whose most sophisticated clinical services attracts patients from all over the country. For this purpose, in 1977, CHC created as one of its many departments, a special unit called the Rural Unit for Health and Social Affairs (RUHSA), which was to be operated by a specialist director under the guidance of a managing committee consisting of CHC staff and outside experts. RUHSA's area of operation covers a block spread over 180 km^2 with a population of around 100 000, living in 84 villages and hamlets, 75 per cent of whose families were living below the poverty line; it is typically one of the last developed blocks of the State.

Within this specific jurisdiction, RUHSA assumed the role of a catalyst for social change, and has been experimenting with its philosophy that 'health is both a means and a measure of development'. Adopting an interdisciplinary approach, it has sought to pursue health and development simultaneously, including education and income-generating activities. In seeking to secure people's involvement in all aspects of its work, it has successfully brought into being an infrastructure of community institutions and volunteers who can respond to the needs and problems of the community, and take leadership in various areas of development. In its operational organization, the role of volunteers drawn from the community has been indispensable. For this purpose the block is divided into 18 units, of which two are Central Service Units (CSUs), and 16 are Peripheral Service Units (PSUs). A PSU serves a population of 5000 to 7000 and a CSU serves a population of 10 000 as well as providing referral services to eight PSUs. Each PSU has five Family Care Volunteers (FCVs), one Health Aide (HA), and one Rural Community Organizer (RCO). Of these, the FCV is the ultimate ground-level worker, looking after the needs of around 200 families; she is trained in simpler medical skills and preventive care. A PSU is assisted by a Village Health Committee. There is a hierarchy of higher-level workers to plan, co-ordinate, oversee, and evaluate the rural health care promoted through the

FCVs, with the active involvement of village committees (Ford Foundation 1987).

The results achieved by RUHSA with this type of management set-up have been remarkable, though more visible in the field of health than in that of rural development. In a brief span from 1978 to 1983, the crude birth rate had decreased from 36 to 24; the crude death rate from 15 to 8; the infant mortality rate from 116 to 65; and the child (1–5 years) mortality rate from 23 to 11. Much of the credit goes to the structure of CHC, the management and training skills at its command, the co-operation it could secure from the Central and State governments, and the goodwill it could build up for itself in the course of the project's tenure. The cost of the project has been on the high side and its replicability is not generally considered to be feasible. There are very few college-hospitals like the CHC and few of them would dirty their hands with rural health.

The second example has adopted quite a different strategy. Rather than extending health services from a referral apex to grass-roots level communities like RUHSA, it starts from below in search of the necessary referral apex; rather than expanding the scope of its health work to encompass rural development, it mounts a development effort which, in due course, internalizes health. Accordingly, it is aptly named 'Action for Welfare and Awakening in Rural Environment', or AWARE (Ford Foundation 1988).

AWARE is an exclusive organization, intended to catalyse self-reliant development among the tribals and the scheduled caste population of the Talangana region of Andhra Pradesh, which is among the most backward areas of rural India. There are 1750 villages in the region, with a population of nearly a million people. AWARE's avowed goal is 'to create self-sustaining rural and tribal communities through a process of their socio-economic and psychological invigoration'. Its focus is people, whose development calls for 'a complex continuum of psycho-socio-economic action'. This is a strategy which necessarily accords health an integral place of great significance.

The idea originated in the mind of its founder-chairman, who relinquished his high-level civil service job for the purpose in 1969. He and his two activist associates, after deep deliberation, finally founded AWARE in 1975. 'The basic strategy of AWARE', it is claimed, 'is to awaken the people, to make them identify their own problems and to prepare them to devise their own solutions and plan for action. The oppressed must not only recognise that they are oppressed but must also be aware of what they can do legally, peacefully and constructively to overcome the oppression.'

The target unit of their operational strategy is the village, a microcosm whose potential for development has remained undermined for a long pauperizing past. AWARE's work in a village, therefore, begins with an attack on the culture of submissiveness of these rural folk through well-tailored educational and organizational programmes. Its three-pronged strategy (generating awareness, creating employment and income-generating opportunities, and ensuring satisfaction of basic needs on an equitable basis) is directed towards the transformation of the present hapless and helpless communities living below subsistence into 'alert, sustainable and autonomous communities and to reach them to a point where they can function on their own steam without further catalyzing help from outside.'

After identifying a target village, AWARE launches its long drawn-out process of awareness creation through informal discussions with individuals and groups, leading ultimately to the formation of a village association. Thereafter, an action plan is drawn up for the comprehensive social, economic, and psychological development of the village. AWARE's activities in this regard last for around seven years. Thereafter it withdraws, and this signifies the community's readiness to be self-reliant and to assert its capacity to act on its own behalf.

Since 1975, AWARE has withdrawn in such a manner from over 200 villages. Promotion of economic growth is launched, while the process of awakening the community is well on its way. These activities include upgrading a variety of agricultural and related operations and rejuvenation of traditional arts and crafts, as well as the introduction of new trades. AWARE's main role here relates to education and training, and to the creation of the necessary organizations, particularly the co-operatives. The third component, relating to minimum needs, operates meanwhile to promote community health, women and child welfare, community reorganization, disaster and cyclone relief, rehabilitation of bonded labour, and legislative assistance to weaker sections. All these are mutually reinforcing and overlapping; their simultaneous operation has contributed to their remarkable success as a package of social development. Health, among these elements of social progress, has been the prime mover in eliciting a positive response from the people, and bringing to AWARE great popularity and goodwill.

AWARE's involvement in community health began with cyclone medical relief during the late 1970s. This was so successful that people insisted that AWARE should continue health work in normal times as well. It therefore agreed to operate clinical services which, the people had pleaded, was their felt need. Over the next decade, it established three Community Health Centres and a Floating Hospital, all of which are very popular and are, in fact, overworked. The services they provide are: medical care, preventive care, health education, training of paramedica and CHWs, nutrition education, environmental sanitation, and leprosy control. In the process of this development, AWARE has created a host of CHWs and propagated among them the notion that 'community medicine (and health) is community development'. Its staff at the lowest level now includes 9900 village health-cum-development workers, 120 village organizers, 99 cluster (a group of 20 villages) development officers, 17 area co-ordination officers, and three zonal officers.

The health work of AWARE has been fairly successful and most remarkable in that it is effectively integrated with the social, economic, and psychological development of the people. Though it began with medical cure, its scope has successively expanded to preventive and promotive health care. The enthusiasm generated among the people for preventive health care is aptly reflected in the following, admittedly inadequate and rather poor translation of a song sung by an old man, who works as a motivator in charge of women health workers.

> In the bottle we lost our health and wealth and pledged our souls
> in bonded labour.
> Then the change came and a desire to right the wrong
> The Awakening which grew from neighbour to neighbour
> In village after village, from neighbour to neighbour
> Leafy vegetables are good, so eat them
> Vaccinations help, so take them
> Without antenatal knowledge and care
> What will come your way are death and despair
> What is leprosy, do you know it is not fatal
> Without proper shots it's tetanus that is lethal
> Avoid the darkness and the loss of life
> Awaken to knowledge that is your birth right.

Weaning away the tribals and the deprived rural folk from the long-ingrained habit of drinking alcohol has perhaps been AWARE's most successful preventive and promotive health work. It is reported that 'the entire *harijan* (scheduled caste) and tribal population in 1,200 out of the 1,750 villages has stopped alcohol consumption and assures that there is no resumption of drinking through stringent collective monitoring'.

The philosophy underlying the concepts of AWARE is appealing, and its operational strategy is imaginative and viable. However, AWARE's role has not gone beyond that of a NGO supplementing the government's effort. It has also depended rather disproportionately on outside funding, though this is vehemently denied by the AWARE activists. It is also alleged that

> much of AWARE's strength is tied up with the personal charisma of its leadership symbolised in the chairman. However, the conviction seems to have settled down deep into all levels of AWARE that the chairman is only one of the links and not the fastener in the human chain that binds AWARE. In the final analysis, the survival of AWARE depends not on the chairman but on the people who are its true *leader*.

It is easy to lionize the people, but 'people' remains an abstraction to which meaning can be imparted only by activists springing up from within, or when committed and self-effacing leadership emerges to shake them from their slumber and put them on the path towards comprehensive and basically self-reliant development. AWARE's target population was fortunate in the farsighted leadership that helped them to mobilize themselves for their own progress in development, which is a correlate, if not a prerequisite, for improvement of the conditions essential for their health. AWARE's job has been to show the light, so that those hibernating in darkness in a state of pauperization may find their way out of poverty, misery, and ignorance.

The Alma-Ata Declaration and PHC

Despite evident differences in their approach to rural health care, both the top-down RUHSA and the bottom-up AWARE use CHWs in their respective jurisdictions. Similarly, the other NGOs operating in different parts of the country also use CHWs, under a variety of designations, and with varying degrees of success. Obviously, there are wide differences in the nature and scope of work done by CHWs, in the niche they occupy in the organization, and in their status *vis-à-vis* other health functionaries. On the whole, it would apear that those CHWs in the voluntary sector perform much better than their counterparts working under the central government's Rural Health Scheme of 1977. Yet there is no evidence anywhere to show that the CHWs' performance is any closer to that expected of them within the system of health care delivery envisaged in the Alma-Ata Declaration of Health for All.

For an idea of the kind of functionary we should have as a CHW within the system of PHC advocated by the Alma-Ata Conference, we may briefly recall here the content of the said Declaration (WHO 1978*a*). Admittedly, it represents the essence of all the world's wisdom on the subject of human health. It pronounces a time-bound goal for universalizing positive health, imparts meaning to the concept of health, and specifies the means for the attainment of the said goal. That goal is the attainment of a level of health that would permit all peoples of the world to lead a socially and economically productive life by the year 2000. While all nations commonly share this august goal, there are great differences of opinion about quantitative indicators of a social state that can be said to represent the attainment of a so qualitatively defined level of health. We need not join this unfruitful debate, beyond insisting that, at the target date, the State should at least be characterized by the universalizaton of easy access to PHC, which is claimed to be a means of attaining the said goal.

The Declaration is in many ways a unique statement of faith. In its very first clause, while bestowing the status of a fundamental human right upon 'health', it imparts to that word the widest possible meaning by adding a mere qualification to it. Health is so qualified as 'a state of *complete* physical, mental and social well-being and not merely the absence of disease or infirmity'. The same clause also asserts that the attainment of the highest possible level of health is a most important *social* goal. Having shifted the onus of attaining Health for All on to society, the Declaration goes on to enjoin the people to exercise their 'right and duty to participate individually and collectively in the planning and implementation of their health care'.

In making these pronouncements of the right, the duty, and the social stake, the Declaration duly recognizes the simultaneous pursuit of the role of individuals (and their families), and that of their immediate society (social organization or community) as one of the basic premises for the attainment of the goal of Health for All. The goal may be said to be contingent, therefore, on two basic requirements: (1) the nature and the level of wholesome development, including unity, integrity, and viability, of the community, and (2) the adequacy and quality of social orientation as well as the level of personal development of its individual members. Thus, the reorientation of both the community and its members is a prerequisite for the creation and successful operation of PHC, which is identified by the Declaration as 'the key to attaining this target as a part of development in the spirit of social justice'.

Having eloquently argued that health is both a right and a duty, individually and collectively enjoyed and exercised, the Declaration goes on to insist that it is imperative to establish, maintain, and monitor a PHC system as the foundation which may support secondary and tertiary referral medical services as required. 'Primary health care', the Declaration pronounces,

> is essential health care based on practical, scientifically sound and socially acceptable methods and technology made universally accessible to individuals and families in the community through *their full participation* and at a cost that the community and country can afford to maintain at every stage of their development in the spirit of *self-reliance* and *self-determination*. It forms an integral part both of the country's health system and of the overall social and economic development of the community. It is the first level of contact of individuals, the family and community with the national health system, and constitutes the first element of a continuing health care process. (WHO 1978*a*)

Leaving aside the traces of equivocation in this long-winded definition of PHC, we may underscore several of the essential features that it must carry in order to deliver positive health successfully, in a spirit of social justice to all members of the community. It is clear that PHC, unpolluted by discrimination of any kind, cannot be a gift to any community from outside; neither the government nor any NGO from outside should be expected to implant the system on to the community. It can only be the creation of the exercise of self-determination by a self-reliant community commanding the full participation of all its members. The quantum and quality of health care the community may give to itself cannot exceed in expenditure the resources it can find from within itself, supplemented by the legitimate entitlement of its share from the country's outlays on national health.

Primary health care is, in other words, a social process of self-reliant satisfaction, by the joint and several effort of the members of a community, of one of its basic needs, to the extent it can afford to do so. It is 'essential health care' as determined by adequate research of factors determining health in the given physical setting and social milieu; it effectively combines promotive, preventive, curative, and rehabilitative aspects of health care; it involves for the community and its members a process of continual 'learning by doing'; its operation extends beyond health to agriculture and animal husbandry, food, industry, education, housing, public works, communications, and related sectors, which need to be carried out in a co-ordinated manner; its self-reliant development and management must make full use of local resources; it must be backed by an adequate referral system of secondary and tertiary medical services, and it must, among other things, rest on trained CHWs as well as reoriented, traditional practitioners.

CHWs and Gandhi's Constructive Workers

The recollection of the high principles and operational mechanics of PHC, despite their universal familiarity within concerned circles, serves only to emphasize the tremendous amount of 'social engineering' that is required to impart necessary cohesion and competence to community organization and to awaken, enthuse, educate, and empower its members to take up this task in their own interest. It is a political process of preparing a people hitherto steeped in ignorance, apathy, and dependence for a free and unfettered exercise of their right and their duty, and, in matters of health, to give them the due which was denied to them for a long time past. The holistic concept of PHC can be made operational at ground-level only through a band of social or community level workers who can enter the minds and hearts of the people whom it must serve.

The question that must be addressed is, what kind of workers do we need for this community level health work, whose scope is so defined as to exhaust the aspects and dimensions of what is loosely called 'development'? There is no ready-made answer to this question in the changed and changing national scene, but if we equate, as we must, this task to that of universalizing human freedom, the worker we need is of the same kind and calibre that M. K. Gandhi created, in the course of the freedom struggle, to take up constructive work as the main means of tranforming India's rural masses into a non-violent force of freedom fighters.

Today, the fight has to be fought against widespread misery, disease, ignorance, superstition, inequity, injustice, and similar ills, which have prevented political freedom from being translated into social and economic freedom for the masses. To develop health is to develop people, which is a task begun quite early by Gandhi in his leadership of the struggle for political freedom. It was, unfortunately, abandoned soon after that freedom was won. It has to be resurrected and refashioned in the light of today's requirements. This is entirely possible, for Gandhi, too, had desired to awaken rural India into an era of self-determination, self-reliance, a measure of self-efficiency, and decentralization of social, economic, and political power; that is, into an era of democratization of freedom, which as yet remains for the power base to profess as a national goal.

Gandhi's 'Constructive Programme' (CP) was based on as thorough an understanding of the state of the Indian masses as one could acquire, by entering their hearts and minds and by living a life no better in material terms than that of the poorest of his countrymen. He realized that life in rural India, once known for its cultural exuberance, was, thanks to long-standing colonial oppression, reduced to that characterized by poverty and misery, by death and disease, by servility and submission, by self-abnegation and resignation, not by the will to live but by the sufferance of survival at subhuman levels of existence. He had come back from South Africa, not to lead the small more vocal, educated, *comprador* class in their bid to displace British rule, but to awaken India's teeming millions to their plight, and show them the way to come out of their animal-like state of utter dependence into a life of human self-assertion, self-reliance, and self-determination. He agreed that political freedom might greatly facilitate his task of enlisting the participation of the masses in their own economic, social, and moral progress, but he was convinced that to lift the people up from the depth of their degradation could not be deferred until the conquest of colonialism.

He therefore designed his CP in order to help the people to help themselves to improve their lot. He conceded that the CP could be a drill for a non-violent fight for freedom, but he insisted that, if pursued throughout the countryside with total commitment and untiring zeal, it would build the nation up in such a way that autocratic rule of any kind would vanish without any struggle whatsoever. The CP, as a whole, was meant to free the human spirit of a nation of some 400 million, which knew no bounds and bonds. It was meant to lead the people from darkness into light and from death to life-eternal.

There are as many as 18 items of social work in the CP designed by Gandhi for the social transformation of rural India (Gandhi 1945). Health *per se* forms one of the most crucial elements of this transformation. What is much more striking is the fact that this package of measures of rural reconstruction represents a ready-made recipe for the kind of action programme that should be taken up for the attainment of positive health by the people. This is not surprising, for the Alma-Ata Declaration not only approaches health in a holistic manner, but proceeds to encompass, within the fold of its conception of PHC, political, economic, social, and environmental correlates of health. The health of the people was, for Gandhi, both an end and a means for rural progress; similarly, the Alma-Ata Declaration did not advocate the improvement of health only for its own sake, but also as a means that permitted people to lead a socially and economically productive life. While it does not acknowledge it in so many words, the Alma-Ara Declaration may be said to rediscover Gandhi's CP.

Let us, in any case, consider the 18 items in Gandhi's package for their relevance for progress in the field of people's health. All these items directly or indirectly impinge on the state of people's health, but the implications of each of them for health are not self-evident—hence the need for this brief reference. Each of the items may be positioned in a manner that may make it appear to belong to several fields of social endeavour; without attaching too much importance to this complexity, we may, for the sake of convenience and brevity, list the items under the following headings:

Health proper

- Inculcation in the minds of individuals of the rules and habits of attaining and maintaining good health
- Prohibition of the use of alcohol and other intoxicants

- Village cleanliness and environmental sanitation
- Treatment of lepers and leprosy control

Education

- Adult and Continuing education
- Basic education suited to the requirement of rural India
- Role of students and their reorientation away from the dependency-creating western education in favour of the one suited to the needs and the genius of their age-old culture

Economy

- Khadi; that is, the Swadeshi movement emphasizing maximum utilization of production based on labour and resources
- Village industries, including rejuvenation of old arts, crafts, and handcrafts, and the establishment of appropriate modern small scale processing units
- Uplift of farmers
- Welfare of farm labourers in particular, and all labourers in general
- Economic equity informing all social and economic relations

Society

- Communal unity and harmony
- Removal of untouchability; that is, of discrimination based on caste, class, and ethnicity, in all its forms
- Welfare of tribal people
- Emancipation of women, leading to equality of status between men and women

Communication

- Development of the national language
- Promotion at the same time of different mother tongues.

The above package indeed represents a minimum programme if the derelict rural people have to acquire the capability to build up for themselves a suitable PHC system on their own, in a spirit of social justice and self-determination. The unit of Alma-Ata's PHC, as well as of Gandhi's CP, is the village community, which must function as a dynamic social organization capable of invoking the active participation of all its members in the interest of *Sarvodaya*;

that is, economic, social, and moral progress for all, without any exception.

In the establishment of PHC, or in the transformation of rural society, the pivotal role has to be played by the CHW, or the Constructive Worker fashioned in the Gandhian mould.

From the mid-1920s onwards, Gandhi had promoted interest among his followers to take up constructive work; often he pursuaded those of his followers whom he found particularly suitable to take up specific items of the CP as their specialization. A Constructive Worker was, as a rule, left free to choose any of the 18 items to begin with, but it was understood that he would be required in the course of time progressively to expand the scope of his work to cover other items as well.

During his lifetime, Gandhi created a large cadre of Constructive Workers, covering more than 10 000 village communities in different parts of the country. They were fairly successful in spreading social consciousness and political awareness among the people for whom they worked. They were all catalysts of social change; their task was not to investigate or even promote change, but to awaken people to their plight, and enable them to redress it on the basis of their own strength. They were men of high moral character; they were worldly-wise, but not highly learned; they were committed to the cause, but not for personal profit or goodwill; they were adept in setting an example by leading a self-reliant life of dignity and simplicity verging on penury; they were selfless and even self-effacing. They were, in short, the torch-bearers hidden in the shadows of their torches, lighting the path of progress for the people they sought to serve.

The Constructive Workers received no formal training beyond their own internalization of Gândhi's wayward ways of serving the poor, the miserable, and the wretched of this ancient land. Determined to participate in the regeneration of rural India, they made their home among the most deprived of these people, to share their deprivations and teach them how to overcome them. Since all the miseries of their existence translated themselves ultimately into a high incidence of morbidity, mortality, and stunted growth of both persons and personalities, every Constructive Worker was required to carry with him a spinning wheel, as a symbol of ways to fight poverty, together with a broom, a basket, and a pickaxe as means of removing the disease-causing wretchedness of their surroundings.

It may be argued, thus, that the Constructive Worker of Gandhi's creation was, at the least, a complete CHW. Unfortunately, since his passing away, Constructive Work has been pushed into hibernation. At long last, Alma-Ata has provided the opportunity for its resumption and it is appropriate that the resumption should begin with the field of health.

CONCLUSION

The speculation on the feasibility of the goal of 'Health for All by 2000' can therefore end on a positive note, by asserting that the feasibility rests with the adoption of the time-tested constructive approach to rural health. We believe that, in this regard, CHWs must play the same role as the Constructive Workers played in rural reconstruction in the face of the constraints imposed by colonial rule.

How they may now, in a more congenial atmosphere of independence, organize and pursue their work may be illustrated by the lessons drawn from the experience of one of the oldest Constructive Work institutions, which has worked for the uplift of one of the most deprived of the groups in the country's population, the *Adivasis* or the tribals of South Gujarat, one of whom has adorned the Chief Ministership of his State. These lessons are presented to telling effect in a small booklet by a leader and a teacher of Constructive Workers, who spent almost the whole of his active public life in the same place (Dave 1960).

The author posits in a Constructive Worker the virtues and skills of a teacher specialized in non-formal, continuing education. He also assumes that the Constructive Worker comes from outside to adopt a village community, in whose people he must seek to lose his own identity. From the vast experience of his own interactions with, and training of, numerous successful workers, he has concluded that the best way to begin Constructive Work in a community, whose members are unfamiliar to him, is for the Worker to start by organizing village children into *balwadis* (pre-school nurseries). This is the counterpart of similar, but indifferently run, institutions officially sponsored under what is called the Intensive Child Development Scheme. From here, the Worker should proceed to organize residential schools for boys and girls, and then to the informal education and training of out-of-school older boys working as cowherds. He suggests a highly imaginative and attractive programme of imparting knowledge and skills to this group, which was found to be the most receptive.

Next, he suggests village cleanliness, including maintenance of spotless roads, lanes, and bylanes, the cleansing of wells and drains, and the maintenance of hygienic and harmless latrines. Then follows the organization of a village health centre. In this regard he warns the Constructive Worker against assuming the role of a doctor, though he may administer commonly known remedies for easily identifiable common ailments. However, he calls upon the Worker to acquire the knowledge and skills of nursing; of the purification of drinking water; of the cleanliness of residences, clothes, and surroundings; of occupational health; of dealing with unhealthy habits and thought and behaviour; and of the observation of restraints and discipline in life. For the rest, he discusses in detail the content and methodology of pursuing programmes for the economic self-reliance and self-sufficiency of the village; for people's (mainly adults') education; for the organization of a village volunteer corps; for interactions with nearby towns and cities; and the imperative for the Worker to remain completely self-reliant.

This is but one recipe for the grooming and guidance of a CHW, and there are many others. In all cases, the burden of their advice is that the attainment of health by rural people is necessarily very closely interrelated with diverse fields of development. This calls for a committed, self-effacing CHW, who need not be highly educated, but who will benefit from training in social or community welfare work, if not in the sophisticated operations of what is unhelpfully termed as social engineering.

6

Community Health Workers in Tanzania

H. K. HEGGENHOUGEN AND
F. M. MAGARI

INTRODUCTION

Tanzania has a well-earned and long-standing reputation for having developed a comprehensive health care policy, and for attempting to make basic, primary health care (PHC) services available to its total population in both rural as well as urban areas. Already in 1978, 92 per cent of the population were within 10 km, and 70 per cent were within 5 km of a health facility. In 1988, the slightly higher proportion of 72 per cent of the population were within 5 km of such a facility. Despite this extraordinary effort to construct an equitably distributed health facilities infrastructure it is, however, still the case that of the country's approximately 8500 villages there are some 5000 without a formal health facility. More than 20 years ago, as now, it was felt that community health workers (CHWs) or *wahudumu wa afya vijijini* could be trained and deployed in village health posts (VHPs), to provide curative and preventive care at village level, and to assist and complement services provided at the formal government facilities. Both the government, through the Ministry of Health, and voluntary agencies, and a number of donor agencies (for example, UNICEF, DANIDA, NORAD, SIDA) in different regions of the country, are involved in training and supporting CHW programmes.

Tanzania has been a leader in this decision of extending health services to all its people, and to utilize CHWs in isolated rural communities as one means of doing so. The example set by Tanzania in this area has received wide publicity, especially through the film *A fair share of the little we have*, and through the extensive readership of the chapter, *Meeting basic health needs in Tanzania*

(Chagula and Tarimo 1975) in the well-known WHO book, *Health by the people* (Newell, 1975).

Originally, when the first government CHW efforts were initiated in 1969, the CHWs were seen as temporary workers providing services in villages where subsequently a dispensary would be established. It was soon realised, however, that it was, and still is, unrealistic to think in terms of a dispensary for every village in the foreseeable future. The view that the training and deployment of CHWs is a stop-gap measure has now changed, and the CHWs are being recognized, and often valued, as permanent village-based PHC workers, who are integral members of their own communities, but who also have, at the very least, an informal relationshp with the official government health services.

Two major studies on CHWs have been carried out in Tanzania. The most recent of these was conducted by the Tanzanian Ministry of Health (AFYA) in 1987–88 (AFYA 1989), and the earlier study was the CHW Research and Evaluation Project, jointly carried out by AFYA/Muhimbili Medical Centre, the London School of Hygiene and Tropical Medicine and NORAD in 1980–83 (Heggenhougen *et al.* 1987). The material for this chapter is primarily derived from the results of these two studies.

HEALTH AND DEVELOPMENT IN TANZANIA

A primary emphasis in the constitution of the Tanganyika African National Union—TANU (which in 1977 merged with the Zanzibari Afro Shiraz party to form the ruling Chama Cha Mapinduzi–CCM), even prior to Independence in 1961, was that the aim of the new government should be to 'mobilise all natural resources towards the elimination of poverty, ignorance and disease' (Nyerere 1968:14). Despite this commitment, however, the health services did not change much during the first few years of Independence, during which the emphasis was placed on other sectors, and within the health sector almost exclusively on the maintenance and expansion of curative services in urban areas. During the 1961–64 Development Plan period health was allocated 4 per cent of the national budget. Of course, the health budget has never exceeded twice that proportion, and in 1986–87 it was down to 3 per cent, as shown in Table 6.1.

Initially, the demands of urban elites had a great influence on

Table 6.1 The health budget share of the total Government expenditure 1970–86

Financial year	Total Tanzanian budget (mill. Tsh)	% change	Health budget (mill. Tsh)	% change	% of total budget	Health budget share % change
1970–71	2925		152		5.2	
1971–72	2465	17	158	4	6.4	23
1972–73	3081	29	203	28	6.6	3
1973–74	4081	32	362	78	8.9	35
1974–75	6065	49	416	15	6.9	−22
1975–76	6241	2	430	3	6.9	—
1976–77	7843	26	522	21	6.7	−3
1977–78	8195	4	649	24	7.9	18
1978–79	12 650	54	723	11	5.7	−28
1979–80	13 809	9	769	6	5.6	−2
1980–81	16 383	19	864	12	5.3	−5
1981–82	16 632	2	926	7	5.6	6
1982–83	18 993	14	1014	7	5.3	−5
1983–84	22 615	19	946	−7	4.2	−20
1984–85	24 680	9	977	3	4.0	−5
1985–86	30 458	23	1273	30	4.2	5
1986–87	55 595	83	1693	33	3.0	−29

Source: AFYA/SIDA 1987:123.

health policy (Segal 1973) but the lack of trained manpower also inhibited the rapid change in the character of the health care system. During these early years it was mainly left to the missions and the so-called Native Authorities (renamed Local Authorities) to concentrate on rural health services.

Because of the recognized inconsistency between the stated goal of the government and actual practice during the first years of the new government, the Titmuss Committee was formed to make recommendations for practical changes within the health system. The resulting Titmuss Report (Titmuss *et al.* 1964) does, in fact, mark a watershed in the development of health services in Tanzania. As a result of the report the 1964–69 Development Plan emphasized, and specifically outlined, rural health care and preventive

Table 6.2 Rural/urban government health expenditures 1971–81

	1971–72	1975–76	1977–78	1980–81
Urban	80%	62%	60%	58%
Rural	20%	38%	40%	42%

Source: AFYA 1982:35.

services development, and called for (1) greater attention to be placed on preventive services; especially in the rural areas; (2) co-ordination between mission and government services, and (3) the construction of more rural health centres and dispensaries. A definite start was made during this period, but both because of limited resources for construction of facilities as well as curative oriented health manpower training, the goals were not achieved as completely as expected.

The Arusha Declaration in 1967 was yet another attempt to emphasize socialist policies for the benefit of the total population, and had a great impact not only within Tanzania but internationally, as a policy widely discussed for possible emulation elsewhere. The government nationalized the means of production, and the resultant increased resources were to be used for the needs of the nation through development efforts which focused on education, provision of clean water, and curative and preventive health services. *Ujamaa* (familyhood) villages were also instituted, based on the philosophy of sharing available resources, collective economic work, and self-reliance. Much has been written on the *ujamaa* villages and on self-help in Tanzania, and it is fair to say that the reality has not always been what was expected (Nyerere, 1968, 1972; Tarimo 1978). But, although the reality has not always lived up to the stated ideal, a definite shift can be seen to have taken place since the late 1960s, and during the 1970s, in terms of an increasing proportion of the health budget being devoted to rural as well as to preventive services (Table 6.2).

The number of health personnel also increased markedly, especially those working in rural areas (Table 6.3), and the increase in the numbers of dispensaries and health centres was outstanding (Table 6.4).

The health statistics have also improved since Independence, with a shift in life expectancy from 35 years in 1961 to 50 years in

Table 6.3 Urban/rural distribution of staff

	1972	1976	1978	1980
Doctors				
urban	418	487	513	598
rural	216	399	479	547
Nurses				
urban	2606	2760	2868	3570
rural	1653	2060	3322	4705
Medical auxiliaries (MAs and RMAs)				
urban	208	456	624	910
rural	605	1363	2166	2800

Source: AFYA 1982:35).

1980, for example, and a decrease in the infant mortality rate (IMR) from 160 in 1000 in 1967 to 137 in 1000 in 1978. Such improvements are, of course, not necessarily a direct reflection of the increase in preventive and rural health care services, although a good case can be made for saying these improving statistics do reflect the overall development efforts of the country.

Despite the impressive infrastructure of health facilities in Tanzania, it still remains that the majority of villages do not have even a dispensary, and though such a facility may be only 10 km away, even this distance has been seen to be a definite impediment to

Table 6.4 Development of rural health care infrastructure 1961–80

	1961	1972	Actual 1980	Target 1980
Health centres	22	99	239	300
Dispensaries	975	1501	2600	2300
Medical assistants	200	335	1400	1200
Rural medical aides	380	578	2310	2800
MCH aides/village midwives	400	700	2070	2500
Health assistants	150	290	681	1800

Source: AFYA 1982:19.

Table 6.5 Type of health facilities according to administrative areas

Administrative area	No.	Type of health facility	No.
Villages	8300+	Village health posts	2000?
Wards	1963	Dispensaries	2600
Divisions	360	Health centres	239
Districts	104	District and rural hospitals	126
Regions	20	Regional hospitals	17
Zone	4	Consultant hospitals	3
		Special hospitals	2

Source: AFYA 1979, except for VHPs.

utilization. The training and use of CHWs have therefore remained an integral part of the country's health sector development policy.

COMMUNITY HEALTH WORKERS, THE TANZANIAN HEALTH CARE SYSTEM, AND VILLAGE ORGANIZATION

Although not official members of the health care services as such, CHWs can be considered the first level of care within a six-tiered health care system, which starts from the VHPs and ends with the consultant and specialist hospitals. These levels of health care generally correspond to the different administrative levels within the country (Table 6.5).

Since a further policy of decentralization (to that implemented in 1972) was established in 1984 each district is now responsible for, and has control over, the health centres and dispensaries within its domain, including budget allocations. This obviously fosters a greater sense of self-reliance and an ability to focus on locally defined needs, but it may also result in differences in priority given to the health sector, as well as differences due to differing financial resources, between districts. This situation obviously affects the CHWs and the VHPs as they relate to, and are dependent upon, the staff and resources of the dispensary and/or health centre nearest their own communities. The CHWs are, of course, also linked with the political and administrative structure at ward and division level, as well as with that in their own communities.

Within each Tanzanian village there is a 25-member village council which is elected by the assembly of all (male and female) village adults. The council has five village committees: (1) on production and marketing; (2) on security and defence; (3) on works and transport; (4) on finance and planning, and, (5) on education, culture, and social welfare, with a subcommittee for health. It has been suggested that a separate, sixth, committee should be established for health (Fig. 6.1).

The CHWs are usually members of the village council and of the committee dealing with health. Each village (council) has a chairman, who is sometimes also the head of the village branch of the CCM (political party), and many villages also have a paid village manager to handle their affairs. All villages are sub-divided into ten-household units, headed by a 'ten-cell' leader, or *balozi*. In terms of preventive and promotive work the CHWs will usually need to work quite closely with the chairman and the *balozis*, as well as with the leaders of the women's organizations and, of course, with religious and specially recognized opinion leaders.

THE HISTORY OF CHWs IN TANZANIA

The predecessors to the present CHWs were the paramedical cadres, 'military inspectors', 'dispensers', and 'tribal dressers', who began training in 1926. These health workers were, of course, also the forerunners of the more highly trained health personnel such as the medical assistants, health assistants, and rural medical aides. These personnel, who were all African, were trained to work in rural areas since, except for mission workers, no European professionals wanted to work outside the towns.

It was in the late 1960s, after the events of both the Titmuss Commission Report and the Arusha Declaration, that CHWs began to be trained as such, especially since it was recognized that not even a dispensary would be available for many years to come in most of the newly established *ujamaa* villages. Despite the official policy and encouragement to train such workers, which included official guide-lines, there was little co-ordination as to how these workers were actually selected, trained, and deployed. Selection, training, and subsequent contact and supervision of CHWs greatly depended on the interest, and time, of the District Medical Officer

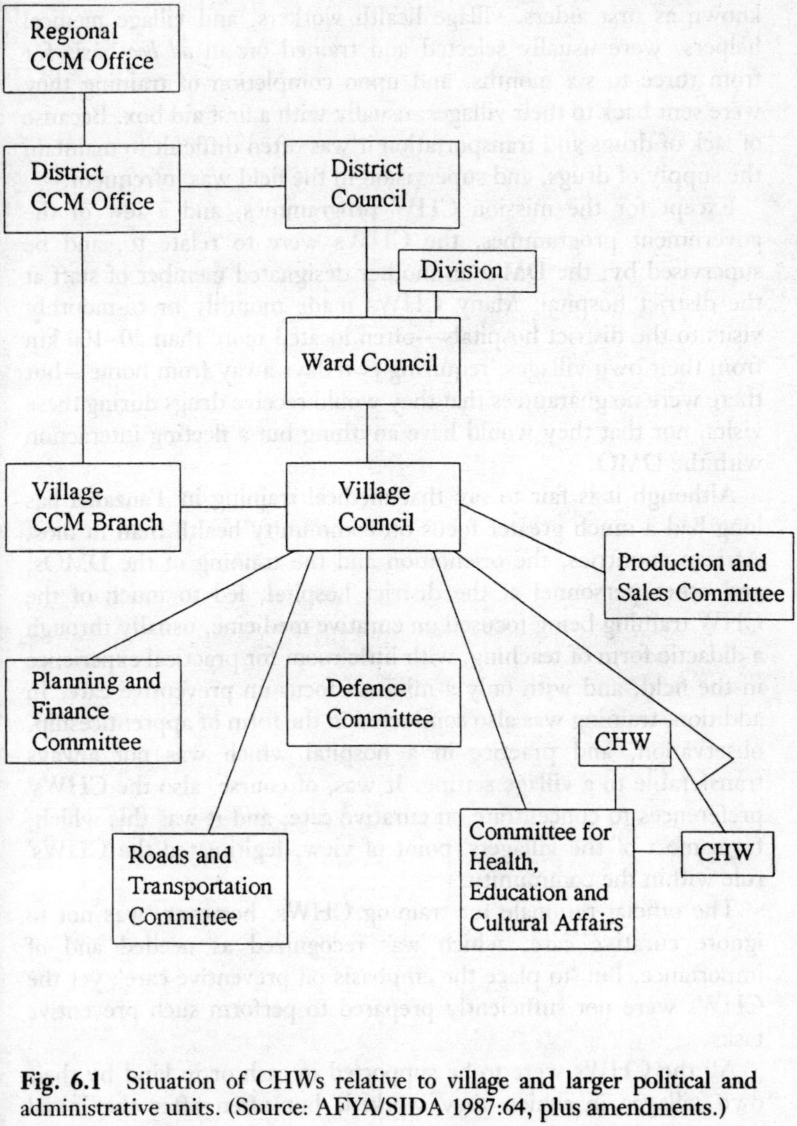

Fig. 6.1 Situation of CHWs relative to village and larger political and administrative units. (Source: AFYA/SIDA 1987:64, plus amendments.)

(DMO), key hospital staff who usually did not remain in any one place more than two years, and on different mission health personnel. Thus, there was a distinct lack of uniformity between CHW programmes in different parts of the country.

The early CHWs of the late 1960s and early 1970s, variously known as first aiders, village health workers, and village medical helpers, were usually selected and trained on an *ad hoc* basis for from three to six months, and upon completion of training they were sent back to their villages, usually with a first aid box. Because of lack of drugs and transportation it was often difficult to maintain the supply of drugs, and supervision in the field was infrequent.

Except for the mission CHW programmes, and a few of the government programmes, the CHWs were to relate to, and be supervised by, the DMO or another designated member of staff at the district hospital. Many CHWs made monthly or bi-monthly visits to the district hospitals—often located more than 50–100 km from their own villages, requiring two days away from home—but there were no guarantees that they would receive drugs during these visits, nor that they would have anything but a fleeting interaction with the DMO.

Although it is fair to say that medical training in Tanzania has long had a much greater focus on community health than in most African countries, the orientation and the training of the DMOs, and other personnel at the district hospital, led to much of the CHW training being focused on curative medicine, usually through a didactic form of teaching, with little room for practical experience in the field, and with only a minimal focus on preventive care. In addition, training was also conducted in the form of apprenticeship, observation, and practice in a hospital which was not always transferable to a village setting. It was, of course, also the CHWs' preferences to concentrate on curative care, and it was this which, from most of the villagers' point of view, legitimated the CHWs' role within the community.

The official rationale for training CHWs, however, was not to ignore curative care, which was recognized as needed and of importance, but 'to place the emphasis on preventive care'; yet the CHWs were not sufficiently prepared to perform such preventive tasks.

All the CHWs were to be supported in cash or in kind by their own villages in which they worked, but often after the initial enthusiasm had died down—and the CHWs had run out of the drugs which they could not replace—not many were supported regularly. This, and the fact that initially a majority of young single men had been trained in town centres, led to a relatively high drop-out rate, with many seeking work in urban areas.

In an intensive follow-up survey in 1982, of 91 CHWs in 58 villages in Handeni District, Tanga Region, 39 active and 15 inactive CHWs were found in their villages, with another 37 having moved away, of which only six were said to be still active as CHWs (Heggenhougen *et al.* 1987:42). Such a drop-out rate (51 per cent) appears to have been the norm rather than the exception. Despite the relatively high drop-out rate estimated for the country as a whole, due mainly to lack of financial support, inadequate supply of drugs, and isolation due to insufficient supervision, by 1983, it was estimated that at least 2000 CHWs were still relatively active throughout the country.

As already mentioned, in addition to the CHWs training in the government programmes, a number of missions, or voluntary agencies, had extensive experience with CHWs. The most well known of these voluntary agencies' efforts were the Hanang, the Mvumi, and the Simavi projects.

The Hanang Project, in Hanang District, Arusha Region, had trained 168 CHWs for 84 villages by 1982 in a training programme that lasted two years. This project had had a relatively low CHW drop-out rate by the time the USAID supported agency handed the project over to the government health system in 1983. It was clear that even though the majority of the two years of practical village-based and classroom training focused on preventive care, the longer the CHWs remained active the greater proportion of their work was spent on curative activities.

The Mvumi Project in Dodoma Region trained CHWs to work within a comprehensive maternal and child health (MCH) and nutrition programme. By 1982, 70 CHWs had been trained, but only half of these were active at that time—only four years after training.

The Simavi Project, started with outside Dutch funding in 1978, functions in two districts in Tanga Region, and also focuses on MCH and nutrition activities, in addition to training and deploying CHWs. The early training only lasted three weeks, but this was later lengthened. The supervision of this project has been extensive,

Table 6.6 Summary of 1053 CHWs in 71 districts in 1982*

1. *Where trained*	%
District hospital	64
Health centre	6
Health cente and dispensary	6
Health centre and district hospital	17
Dispensary and district hospital	6
Villages and various health units	1
2. *Duration of training*	
Less than 3 months	42
3–5 months	21
6 months or more	34
Unknown	3
3. *Further in-service training*	
Further training	28
None	65
Unknown	7
4. *Proportion still active*	
A quarter or less	34
A half	28
Three-quarters or more	32
Unknown	6
5. *Supervised by*	
District Medical Officer	41
Medical assistant or rural medical aide	39
None	10
Unknown	10

* This is almost certainly an underestimate since some DMOs did not know the number of active CHWs.

Source: Heggenhougen *et al.* 1987:40.

but the drop-out rate has still been high (Muhondwa 1982). Table 6.6 provides an overview of the results on training, and supervision, and how many of those trained were active in the 71 districts covered by a study in 1982.

Based on the experience with CHWs up until 1982, and deriving from the 1983 'Guidelines for the implementation of the PHC programme in Tanzania' (AFYA 1983), a concerted effort was made to learn from past mistakes and to rejuvenate the CHW programme within a more uniform training and supervisory system. A six-month curriculum was established to be followed throughout the country, with CHWs trained in special training centres and 'folk development colleges', instead of primarily in the district hospitals, and with at least a third of the training to consist of practical work in the CHWs' own villages or at special training sites. A man and a woman were to be trained for each village, and more mature and married people were to be selected than those previously trained. Supervision was to be handled from the nearest health centre rather than the district hospital. Although the CHWs were still not to be considered a part of the official government system, it was suggested that the government would join with the village communities in providing minimal financial support for the CHWs. Because of lack of government resources this has still not taken place.

In 1983 an essential drugs programme was initiated in Tanzania, with primary support from DANIDA and UNICEF. This programme has significantly improved the availability of required drugs for the major common health problems treated at dispensary and health centre level. It was also foreseen that the CHWs would be included within the essential drugs programme, and it was planned that this should be realized by 1991, by which time an accurate system of obtaining an overview of the total number and location of CHWs in the country should have been realized.

The 1983 guide-lines specified nine tasks to be performed by the CHWs

1. To educate and guide the villagers in matters of health through practical demonstrations in collaboration with village leaders.

2. To demonstrate to villagers methods of food production, storage, and preparation, as well as proper nutrition.

3. To identify and enlighten villagers on those cultural aspects which are detrimental to health.

4. To provide services for mothers and children in collaboration with the traditional birth attendants.

5. To provide curative and preventive services in collaboration with the traditional healers.

6. To manage a village health post in the village.

Table 6.7 Characteristics of CHWs in 1982 and 1988

	1982	1988
Age of CHWs		
Below 20 years	28%	7%
20–29 years	50%	61%
30+ years	22%	32%
Marital status		
Married	48%	78%
Unmarried	52%	22%
Where trained		
Dispensary, health centre, or folk development colleges	36%	91%
Hospitals	64%	9%

Source: AFYA 1989 and Heggenhougen *et al.* 1987.

7. To collect, analyse, utilize, and report health and health-related information.
8. To evaluate health activities.
9. Home visiting.

In addition to the support from, and referral to, the nearest health centre, the CHWs were also to work in relation to specially established PHC co-ordinating committees, established at village, ward, division, district, regional, and national level.

Since 1983, more than 2000 CHWs—a man and a woman for each village—have been trained within the new training programme in all 20 regions of the country. Some of those trained have been previously 'active' and inactive CHWs who have now been retrained and entered into the new supervisory system, but a number of the 2000+ CHWs found active in 1983 have not gone for such re-training, thus making the conservative estimate of the current total number of CHWs in Tanzania at more than 3000. Table 6.7 makes it clear that certain changes have occurred in the characteristics of CHWs between 1982 and 1988.

COMMUNITY HEALTH WORKER EVALUATION

A number of evaluations have been carried out on CHWs in Tanzania. Many of these have been of specific programmes functioning within one or two districts, often conducted by voluntary agencies. Of note in this regard is the substantial study carried out by Muhondwa (1982) of the Simavi Project in Tanga Region.

The evaluations carried out by the Hanang Project, in Arusha Region, are probably some of the more comprehensive of the studies done by voluntary agencies and provided valuable lessons for efforts in other districts, as well as for the country as a whole. As with most of such evaluations, however, they have not been published and are therefore not easily accessible.

In terms of countrywide studies, there have been two major national evaluations of CHWs in Tanzania worthy of note. One of these was the Applied CHW Research and Evaluation Project carried out between 1980–83 (Heggenhougen *et al.* 1987). The other major national evaluation effort was essentially carried out by the Ministry of Health from November 1987 through April 1988, and focused on the efforts initiated since the beginning of 1983, when the national CHW training was rejuvenated largely as a result of the commitment derived from the publication of the PHC Guidelines (AFYA, 1983).

The 1980–83 evaluation used a variety of methodological approaches, from in-depth interviewing and case-study presentations to the use of survey questionnaires. The following are some of the sub-projects included: (1) two surveys of DMOs (in 1980 and in 1982); (2) survey of voluntary agencies; (3) five village case studies; (4) in-depth interviews with (344) CHWs in 23 districts; (5) record of weekly activities of 48 CHWs in 14 districts; (6) inventory of drugs and equipment in 81 village health posts (VHPs) in 15 districts; (7) survey of (654) health service staff and of (87) government officials; (8) village household studies in two districts; and (9) review of CHWs' diagnostic and treatment skills.

The findings of this evaluation may be summarized as follows:

Villagers' perception: Villagers do not usually have a clear idea of the job description of CHWs. Villagers are primarily interested in curative services and unless such services are forthcoming they will not be too interested in preventive activities, nor provide support for the CHWs.

Curative and preventive activities: It is clear that CHWs were most interested in providing curative services and this was also the major interest of villagers, but because of lack of drugs, training, and programme emphasis on preventive care, such services were not always forthcoming. This led to frustration on the part of both the CHWs and of the villagers. It was concluded that '. . . the ability to implement preventive activities may quite directly depend on and can only follow from, the competent provision of curative services'.

Diagnostic and treatment skills: It was generally felt that this was quite poor, yet prior to 1982 no study had been carried out on this. From a small pilot study in Maswa District in May–July 1982, it was shown that CHWs may be able to diagnose simple ailments relatively accurately. However, their knowledge and skills in treating these ailments were poor in terms of prescription of appropriate drugs and drug dosages.

Drugs at the VHPs: From an inventory carried out at 81 VHPs in 15 districts it was shown that about 75 per cent of the VHPs had aspirins and chloroquin tablets and 59 per cent had sulphadimidine, although the available quantities of these drugs were often very small. Less than a third of the VHPs had any other drugs at all (see Table 6.8).

Community expectations and experiences: In general, villagers were in favour of having CHWs, but felt that they should be able to provide more sophisticated curative services. Most eventually wanted a dispensary to be established in their village. Because of the inadequacy of the curative services, according to the villagers, they could not see the importance of what the CHWs did and, in fact, quite a large number of villagers did not really know what they did, and many had not been involved in selecting a CHW for training. If CHWs are to receive community support then they must be of recognizable value to their communities. If self-help activities are to succeed, then these activities must be planned and approved in collaboration with the villagers themselves, and must be recognized as being of some value to them.

Table 6.8 Percentage of VHPs with recommended drugs and items of equipment (81 VHPs in 15 districts)

Recommended drugs	Percentage of VHPs with drug or item
Aspirin tablets	77
Chloroquine tablet	73
Sulphadimidine	59
Mist kaolin	32
Tincture benzoic compound	32
Oral iron tablets	30
Flavin solution	28
Cough syrup	26
Sulphacetamide eye ointment	25
Gentian violet paint	23
Multivite tablets	23
Savlon lotion	20
Lysol	14
Cascara	12
Vitamin B complex tablets	12
Cetrimide lotion	9
Benzyl benzoate emulsion	7
Liniment alba	6
Liquid paraffin	2
Gamaxene powder	1
Other drugs	
Chloramphenicol	16
Magnesium trisilicate	11
Ephedrine	11
Aminophylline	10
Ascorbic acid	9
Eusol solution	7
Piriton tablets	6
Folic acid	4
Carminative mixture	4
Iodine solution	4
Expectorant sedative	4

Note: The inventory form only contained names of drugs which were supposed to be available at the VHPs, but other drugs were also specifically mentioned as being present at some of the VHPs.

Source: Heggenhougen *et al*. 1987:89.

Table 6.9 Visits by health services staff within the previous three months

No visit	53%
Visited at least once by staff from:	
Dispensary	17%
Health centre	12%
District hospital	9%
Division/ward health office	3%
Other	6%

Source: Heggenhougen *et al.* 1987:99.

Supervision and support: Less than half of the 344 CHWs interviewed had had a supervisory visit during the previous three months (see Table 6.9). Only a third of these CHWs reported that they received some financial support from their villages, and only half of these again said that such support was provided on a regular basis. Lack of financial support was the major concern of CHWs, and the chief reason why many of them quit their work.

CHWs and government health services: Most AFYA staff were familiar with CHWs and many had been involved in their training. Although AFYA staff claimed to know what CHWs were meant to do, most emphasized curative tasks. The great majority of AFYA staff felt that CHWs should be a permanent health service cadre. It was clear, however, that the actual working and supervisory relationship of the CHWs with the rest of the health system needed improvement. Reorganization needed to take place to increase the contact of CHWs with dispensaries and health centres, particularly as this related to drug supplies, supervision and continuing education. AFYA staff as well as CHWs, needed training in how to function effectively within a new organizational structure, which facilitated PHC activities and a closer, constructive relationship with CHWs.

The 1987–88 evaluation was carried out in six out of the 20 regions of the country (Arusha, Dodoma, Iringa, Mtwara, Pwani, and Tanga). Ten villages were selected in each of a total of 10 districts (100 villages). Field visits, interviews, and reviews of documents were carried out. Some of the findings of this evaluation are:

Training of CHWs: A definite shift had occurred since 1982 in that the majority of CHW training was now found to be carried out at health centres, dispensaries, or folk development colleges. Although the new CHW curriculum included attention to all eight elements of PHC, curative subjects still constituted a major portion of training, and although the training methods were found appropriate for adults, practical experience was still felt to be insufficient. The length of training is still not uniform, with training ranging from one month to two years, as previously. It was also found that the attempt to enforce the use of a uniform CHW curriculum was inappropriate for every area of the country, since it did not allow for a focus on specific community health problems. In terms of CHW training the evaluation recommendations included and emphasis on:

1. Increased dialogue with the community about the concept of CHWs, especially regarding selection and support.
2. Continued effort to be given to selecting older, mature, settled, and well-motivated candidates for training.
3. The CHW curriculum should be revised to be able to focus on local health needs. Training should emphasize a problem-solving orientation.
4. The training period should not be rigidly defined, but two to three months should be sufficient.
5. Short refresher courses should be held every year.

CHW activities: It was found that most CHWs had a plan of work, but the pattern of work, as in earlier years, remains variable, with nearly half of the CHWs working full-time and the others being part-time workers. Most CHWs still spend the majority of their time on curative activities and in dispensing drugs at the VHPs. This was seen as a result of village demand and of inadequate supervision. When drugs are not available at the VHPs the community will stop financial support of the CHWs. It was noted that CHWs require frequent and regular supervision from the nearest health unit, but this was still usually not forthcoming. Recommendations therefore included a focus on:

1. Emphasizing that supervisors from the nearest health units needed to regularly visit the CHWs.
2. Encouraging village health committees to engage in action against health problems, and to recognize the CHW as an agent of change.

3. The importance of providing the CHWs with a sufficient and regular supply of drugs, especially as this would give credibility to the CHWs.

Drop-outs: It was found that 88 per cent of the CHWs trained since 1983 were still in service at the time of the evaluation in 1988. Those dropping out were usually younger than the rest and often single. At least one reason for this obvious improvement of the situation prior to 1983 may be related to the shift in training of more mature, married, and settled candidates than previously (see Table 6.7), and also that the training took place closer to the CHWs' own villages.

Supervision: It was still found that supervision was inadequate and varied greatly from one district to the next, and there is a relatively low level of involvement of dispensary and health centre staff. Recommendations therefore included:

1. An emphasis in making CHW trainers, at dispensaries and health centres, supervisors of CHWs, and such trainers/supervisors should have participated in making community diagnosis.
2. The need to learn from pilot projects in Bagamoyo and elsewhere on improved ways of supervising and monitoring CHW performance, and to develop such capacities in other districts.

CONCLUSIONS

It was concluded that:

> these findings give a fairly poor impression of the effectiveness of CHWs. Although the conclusions may be doubtful on the diagnostic and treatment capability of the CHWs, it is most probable that the majority of the CHWs in the country are preoccupied with curative care, and that at the same time they suffer from a devastating shortage of drugs. Given this situation it is surprising that as many as 2000 CHWs were still active in 1982, before the new CHW programme started. (Heggenhougen *et al.* 1987:91)

Some of the general recommendations of the 1987–88 evaluation include:

1. Priority to be given to the training of CHW trainers at dispensary and health centre level.

2. The trainers of CHW trainers should include personnel outside the health sector.

3. An emphasis should be made on community diagnosis, community organization, communications, and managerial skills in the curriculum of the trainers of the CHWs.

4. The Centre for Educational Development in Health–Arusha (CEDHA) should develop appropriate health learning materials for the CHW Programme.

The matter of how to support CHWs has still not been solved satisfactorily. It is still questioned whether remuneration should come from the communities or from the government, or from both. It would seem that unless this issue can be resolved the CHW drop-out rates are likely to increase. The Ministry of Health still maintains that the communities must remunerate the CHWs (the government states it cannot afford to do this) and it is also suggested that such government funding, if available, would undermine the basic national philosophy of self-reliance and self-determination. In the villages, however, the question is often raised as to why, in an egalitarian society, villagers should pay for services which are freely available to their urban co-citizens.

It is important to note that the Ministry of Health considers the CHWs 'as critical change agents and as "Torches" in their communities'. Despite the problem of payment, the commitment to CHWs is as firm as ever, since they are seen as an important and affordable way in which to improve universal access to PHC services. What is seen as needed in the future is to revise the CHW curricula to make them relevant to specific problems in different districts, to increase the decentralization of training to the lowest possible level and to solicit 'moral and financial support for the programme from the government, local communities and donor agencies'.

In the wake of the latest CHW evaluation, the Ministry has revised guide-lines for training CHWs. The duration of training has been reduced to two months. Training will be geared towards solving community health and health-related problems through community involvement and multisectoral action. Districts have been given flexibility to adapt guide-lines so as to respond to local needs and demands.

CHWs will be provided with a small list of drugs and essential equipment (as shown in Table 6.10).

Table 6.10 The drug list and equipment for CHWs

Drug list	
Chloroquin tablets	1000
Aspirin/paracetamol	1000
ORS sachets	100
Tetracycline eye ointment 2%	10 tubes
Chloroquin syrup	250 ml
Condoms	400
Ergol tablets	100
Eusol and Flavin can be collected from DMO	
Equipment for CHWs	
First aid kit equipment (for male CHWs)	
Straight scissors	1
Dressing forceps	2
Kidney dish	1
Knife handle	2
Blades	5 packets
Dry cells	4
Clinical thermometer	2
Handbag for the above	1
Torch (flashlight)	1
Dressings per month	
Gauze (1 roll)	1 pound
Cotton wool	1 roll
Bandages (6″ roll)	6
Zinc oxide plaster medium	2 rolls
Tincture of benzoin co.	250 ml
Delivery kit equipment	
Kidney dish	1
Bowl sponge	1
Sheeting plastic	2
Flashlight	1
Scale (25 kg)	1
Surgical scissors (straight)	1
Umbilical cord ligature	100 metres
Fetal scope (wooden)	1
Bag for above equipment	1

The Ministry has also developed two more important documents: the National Health Policy, and the revised PHC strategy. Three of the six objectives contained in these documents are quoted below:

1. To reduce infant and maternal mortality rates and to increase life expectancy through the provision of adequate and equitable MCH services, promotion of nutrition, control of communicable disease, and treatment of common conditions.
2. To sensitize the community on preventable health problems so that the community itself can identify their problems and work out priorities in finding appropriate solutions.
3. To create awareness through family health promotion that the responsibility for one's health rests squarely with the individual as an integral part of the family.

In both the CHW guide-lines and the PHC strategy, Community Based Health Care is given great emphasis. The success of this will depend, among other things, on trained, committed and motivated CHWs. Tanzania now looks set towards rapid expansion and deployment of CHWs, who are regarded as key frontline health workers.

7

The State and democratization in PHC: community participation and the village health worker programme in Zimbabwe

DAVID SANDERS

INTRODUCTION

Political independence came to Zimbabwe in 1980, after many years of bitter struggle by the black majority under the leadership of the nationalist parties against white settler colonial rule. The political situation which had developed during 1979, and which persisted throughout the early post-Independence period, as well as the subsequent ebb in the popular mobilization, sets the context for this case study of village health workers (VHWs).

The chapter is divided into four main sections. The first examines briefly the health situation before Independence, reviewing both the health (or disease) situation and its social context, as well as colonial health services.

The second section, entitled 'The state and popular organization', examines the dynamic evolution of popular involvement in the political process in Zimbabwe, situating this experience within the theoretical discourse surrounding revolutionary transition.

The third section, 'The state, popular organization and health care', is the core of this chapter and comprises five subsections. The first summarizes the major post-Independence changes relevant to health; the second explores the general debate about the nature and role of the VHW in both health care and in mobilizing community involvement, identifying the potential economic and political constraints on such initiatives; the third reviews early developments in VHW schemes in Zimbabwe, both non-governmental and governmental; the fourth subsection examines closely community participation in Zimbabwe's national VHW programme, and the fifth and final subsection charts more recent developments in this area.

The fourth and last section of the chapter concludes and briefly summarizes its main thesis.

HEALTH UNDER COLONIALISM

Patterns of disease

In colonial Zimbabwe, as in other underdeveloped countries, the greatest burden of death and disease fell on infants, young children, and women in the child-bearing period. Furthermore, mortality varied substantially by geographical area, race, and class. In 1980, there was a 1:3.5:10 ratio in infant mortality rate (IMR) between whites, urban blacks, and rural blacks, corresponding to a 39:5:1 ratio in incomes (Ministry of Health 1984*a*). While the IMR of 17 per 1000 for the white population approximated that of the industrialized countries, for the majority black population it was estimated to be 120 per 1000.

Although the better off showed the disease pattern seen in industrialized countries, the majority of the population suffered nutritional deficiencies, communicable diseases, and problems associated with pregnancy. Low birthweight in 10–20 per cent of all births, due mainly to maternal undernutrition and protein-energy malnutrition, were the commonest forms of childhood malnutrition, predisposing the victims to more severe and often fatal infections. The most important of these were measles, pneumonia and tuberculosis—all airborne infections transmitted by respiratory secretions—and diarrhoeal diseases. The latter, along with parasitic diseases, such as schistosomiasis, intestinal worms and certain skin and eye infections, were widespread water-related diseases.

Of the occupational diseases, industrial lung disease such as asbestosis, silicosis (and tuberculosis), and coalminer's lung, together with stress-related disorders such as high blood-pressure and plantation-related problems such as schistosomiasis, malaria, and toxic effects of pesticides and herbicides, were all (and are increasingly) visible but undoubtedly under-reported. Mental ill-health and alcohol-related problems were also common, the latter reflecting itself directly in liver disease and indirectly in sexually-transmitted diseases.

Environmental factors and health

This disease pattern was rooted in the system of production, reproduction, and distribution which prevailed in Rhodesia, reinforced by the structures of racial domination. Undernutrition, which from historical accounts appears to have increased after colonization, was particularly prevalent in the 'Tribal Trust Lands' (TTLs), and among the children of workers on commercial farms. Although the TTLs were termed the 'subsistence sector', with increasing land-alienation and a lack of inputs, many peasants were unable to subsist from agriculture alone. By 1977 they were growing only 60 per cent of the needed amount of the staple maize, reflecting the overcrowding, overstocking, and progressive impoverishment of ecologically unfavourable areas. Endemic malaria further undermined the health of the population in these areas.

Increasingly, families were forced to supplement the unreliable agricultural production with cash remitted from the urban industrial or plantation sectors, while providing a growing supply of landless wage labour, and a dumping ground for aged, diseased, and debilitated workers. Airborne infections spread easily in the cramped, often smoky housing conditions existing in both urban and rural areas. Inadequate water supplies, often distant, and frequently contaminated, predisposed people to common and debilitating intestinal, skin, and eye infections (Ministry of Health 1984*a*).

In the white commercial farming areas, where nearly 20 per cent of the population lived, conditions were often worse. Farm workers experienced extreme income, employment, social, and residential insecurity, particularly if they were of the 40 per cent who had been recruited earlier in the century from Malawi, Mozambique, and Zambia. Living conditions on farms were generally cramped and unhygienic, and access to adequate supplies of safe water and sanitation was rare. With land under private control, and black labourers not recognized in law as 'workers' or residents, neither financial nor legal provision was made for improved working or living conditions. Safety standards were poor for the whole working class, and collective bargaining was undermined by state suppression, high levels of unemployment, and a divided labour movement.

Features of the health care system

These environmental factors undermined much of the impact of the health care system. This system had all the features typical of an inappropriate, inequitably distributed developing country service, compounded by inequalities based on racial discrimination. For example, in 1980–81 the average annual expenditure per head for private sector medical aid society members was $Z144, compared with $Z31 for the urban population using public services and $Z4 for the rural population (Ministry of Health 1984*a*). The latter concealed further disparities, for only districts surrounding urban areas were relatively well served.

There were also disparities in the distribution of health care personnel and in access to facilities. In 1980–81, 44 per cent of publicly funded services went to the urban-based sophisticated central hospitals serving about 15 per cent of the population, while only 24 per cent went to primary and secondary level rural health services for the majority of the population (Ministry of Health 1984*a*).

At Independence, health services in Zimbabwe were being provided by a number of agencies—government, mission, local council, industrial, and private, with the first two being the most important providers for the majority, while private practitioners predominantly catered for the needs of the white minority (Gilmurray *et al.* 1979).

The government health budget in 1979–80 totalled $54.2 million, with 87 per cent being allocated to medical services, of which 31 per cent went to the two central hospitals in the capital, and only 8.3 per cent to preventive services, which were administratively and operationally separated from curative services.

The missions were the most important agency providing health care in rural Zimbabwe. Not only did they provide a medical service for the surrounding population, but they were responsible for the training of most medical assistants before Independence, when the missions functioned (relatively) autonomously. They provided some 30 per cent of the country's total and 66 per cent of all rural hospital beds. Additionally, they cared for 22 per cent of the total number of out-patients, and much of the preventive medical work, particularly antenatal care, childhood growth-monitoring, and immunization, was provided in the rural areas by the missions.

In the large-scale farming areas, health services were extremely poor. Local taxes were collected for road and bridge construction only, and money for schools, clinics and social welfare had to come from beer profits or central government. Hence, rural council clinics were estimated to service 26 000 people each, twice the number in peasant areas (Loewenson 1985).

In line with the distribution of facilities, all categories of health personnel—especially professional grades—were concentrated in the urban areas. In 1980 there were over 1138 doctors, 4652 nurses, 2897 medical assistants, and 393 health assistants. Of the doctors, 42 per cent of those practising in 1981 (900) were wholly engaged in private practice, 80 to 90 per cent of whom were in Harare or Bulawayo. In 1982–83 there were 370 doctors in central and general hospitals, 28 in district and 42 in mission hospitals; that is only about 70, or 5 per cent of those registered to practice, were working in the rural areas (Ministry of Health 1983*a*).

Even the distribution of lower-level 'auxiliaries' (medical assistants) was disproportionately urban, although they and health assistants formed the core of the team at district level and below.

Influence of the struggle for independence

During the last few years of the liberation struggle, and particularly in 1979, health services, especially those provided in the TTLs (predominantly by the missions), were severely disrupted and forced to curtail their operations. Large numbers of rural people, particularly those living in the east and south of the country, were forced into 'protected villages' to isolate them from the guerilla forces. 'Village health workers' were trained in three of the then five provinces to work primarily in these 'protected villages'. However, these workers were self-selected or chosen by the Provincial Medical Officer of Health (PMOH) Staff, with only token approval from the communities in which they were to work.

The academic level set in their training ensured that the average rural dweller was excluded from becoming a VHW. They were trained predominantly in curative work and the training was performed in facilities quite different from those in which they were later to work. They were paid by, and accountable to the PMOH's office. Therefore, as discussed below, these cadres more closely resembled 'auxiliaries' than true CHWs.

At the same time, the liberation forces were training their own health cadres and introducing popular-based health care into the camps and liberated areas of the country. In contrast to the colonial infrastructure, this built community mobilization, participation, and discussion into health care delivery, and developed a mobile and accessible form of care in which the main infrastructure was the people. The challenge at Independence lay in reconstructing and reorganizing a deliberately fragmented, inaccessible, and oppressive form of health care, into one which would serve the needs of all, and respond to changing social and economic demands.

THE STATE AND POPULAR ORGANIZATION

The unfolding relationship, before and after political independence, between the State and the developing institutions of popular organization is crucial for understanding the process of popular involvement or 'community participation'—a process which lies at the heart of both primary health care (PHC) and any CHW scheme.

Features of the revolutionary process

During a period of mass political struggle where an existing state power is being challenged, self-organization of the dominated population in support of the revolutionary process is a frequent occurrence. Specifically, in those situations of substantial challenge to the capitalist state, or in the transition to socialism, the dynamic relationship between the contending 'old' and 'new' State powers is pertinent to a consideration of the Zimbabwean experience.

In his discussion of the transition of socialism and the fate of the capitalist State in the process, Lenin (1976) was quite clear:

> . . . but since the proletariat needs the state as a *special* form of organization of violence against the bourgeoisie, the following conclusion suggests itself: is it conceivable that such an organization can be created without first abolishing, destroying the state machine created by the bourgeoisie for *themselves*.

This certainly does not mean that the socialist revolution can be reduced to insurrectionary action alone and that the real alternative is either 'insurrection' or 'elections'. An insurrection is only the final point of a revolutionary process, and if the relationship of forces is favourable it can be effected practically without casualties, provided the armed apparatus of the capitalist state has first been morally and politically disintegrated, and the legitimacy of workers' and people's councils has been acknowledged by the immense majority of the population, including the soldiers.

It is inconceivable, however, to pass in one fell swoop from the 'normal' state power of the bourgeoisie to the new state power of the workers, supported in underdeveloped countries by the vast majority of the peasants. The transition from one to the other requires time, especially in countries in which the state institutions of bourgeois democracy preserve enormous prestige and legitimacy in the eyes of the majority of workers. The masses must undergo an apprenticeship in new and higher forms of democracy. They must have the time to assimilate the meaning and value of the new state organs they are in the process of creating. At the same time, the institutions of the old regime—above all its armed apparatus—must undergo a process of decomposition and progressive paralysis, without which the *generalized* establishment of the organs of power of the workers and peasants is inconceivable.

The concrete historical stage during which this combined process of decomposition of the capitalist regime and emergence of workers' power occurs, is called the stage of dual power. That is the real 'stage of transition' between the stable state power of the bourgeoisie and the victorious socialist revolution. Dual power is the expression of the class struggle brought to its paroxysm: the struggle between antagonistic state (or pre-state) apparatuses contending for *de facto* power and the allegiance of the majority of citizens over a given territory. Those who dismiss 'dual power' as a situation of the past, unique only to the Russian revolution of 1917, should be reminded that it was repeated in Germany in 1918–19, Northern Italy in 1920, Spain in 1936–37, partially in Chile in 1972–73, Portugal in 1975, and Nicaragua in 1979 (Mandel 1978).

Limited dual power in Zimbabwe

There is some evidence of the existence of the beginnings of a 'dual power' situation in Zimbabwe during the period 1978–81. This situation was most evident in the 'semi-liberated' communal areas, particularly where ZANU (PF) guerrillas had been active for a long period. In these areas the party had created popular organizations, initially responsible for supporting the liberation effort, but later structured to perform essential social and economic tasks as an alternative to the Rhodesian State's rudimentary district administration. In those areas, organizations were made up of various tiers of people's councils, which were set up on village, ward, district, and provincial bases. Functions of these committees at various levels differed considerably; for example, grass-roots village committees dealt with the day-to-day problem of feeding and clothing the guerrillas and providing basic services to the community, while those issues involving the outlay of large sums of money would be passed to higher committees.

Thus in many parts of Rhodesia's rural areas the embryo of a 'new' popular state: one based, to recall Lenin, on 'the direct initiative of the people from below' was in existence. Importantly, these popular structures were allied to *their* army, the guerrilla forces, against the Rhodesian State and army. This alternative embryonic state was, unfortunately, crucially weakened with the Lancaster House Agreement,* and the imposition of the cease-fire, with its effective demobilization of the guerrilla army—the armed wing of the embryonic popular state.

One of the major gains of this revolutionary experience was the practice of direct democracy, where peasants and workers for the first time participated directly in the formulation of policies, and

* A constitutional conference which took place at Lancaster House, London, in late 1979, between the liberation movement (the Patriotic Front), the 'Zimbabwe–Rhodesian' regime and the British Government, defined the terms of Zimbabwe's independence. These included agreement over the post-independence constitution and arrangements to end military hostilities.

their day-to-day implementation and evaluation. Furthermore, the ability of the peasants and workers to control, reject, and re-elect representatives became a reality—a far cry not only from their previous experience, where they had no vote, but even from the experience of those living in western 'democracies', where representatives are elected infrequently to parliament, or local government bodies, without any day-to-day control over their actions being exercised by the electorate who voted them in. This gain has persisted, to some extent, in certain parts of the country, but has been progressively eroded with the passage of time.

However, it cannot be argued that anything more than the *beginnings* of a dual power situation existed in Zimbabwe for a number of reasons. The forms of self-organization created were limited in both their geographical extent and also in their class composition. One of the great weaknesses of the popular struggle was that the working class was never mobilized *as a class*. Of course, a significant fraction of poorer rural dwellers who were actively supporting the liberation struggle could be classified as workers, in the sense that their dominant economic activity involved the selling of their labour power to the mines, plantations, and even to richer peasants. However, the settled workers—the proletariat—were never mobilized, although a considerable degree of militancy and self-organization was manifested in the strike wave which started to sweep the country only two weeks after ZANU (PF)'s crushing victory at the polls, and a month before formal Independence. Nevertheless, far from encouraging, organizing, and channelling the worker militancy towards the development of a dual power situation, the new government expressed its dissatisfaction with workers' actions.

Post-Independence structures and local government

What then of developments since the early days of Independence? What is the basic structure of the post-colonial state, and what is its relationship to popular organization?

Far from being dismantled and supplanted by a decentralized workers' and peasants' state, a centralized hierarchical structure with permanent institutions, the security forces, civil service, judiciary, and so on, has *expanded* since Independence. Not only is the standing army much greater in size, but the civil service has expanded from under 50 000 to 80 000. It is of course true that the *racial* character of the State has changed, but has the essential *class* character of the State changed? Perhaps this question is best answered by looking at the relationship between the present-day state, and the embryonic 'popular state' previously mentioned.

At the time of Independence, it would have been possible—at least in certain geographical areas—to strengthen the existing popular organs by providing them with organizational, financial, and technical support, thus replacing 'officialdom, the bureaucracy, . . . by the direct rule of the people themselves' (Lenin 1976). Although the Lancaster House Agreement, which defined the political and constitutional dispensation at Independence, prevented the dismissal of Rhodesia's civil servants, it did not proscribe the transfer of effective power and decision-making to other institutions, neither did it suggest that the bureaucracy be almost doubled in numbers, nor that a complex system of local government be created.

Between 1980 and 1982, District Councils vested with local administrative development powers were established, replacing the colonial District Commissioners and chiefs. Although this system of local government is a significant advance over the previous structure, with ward representatives elected by popular vote and with greater resources than in the past, it none the less remains an extension of the central state. Full-time local government officials are salaried by and responsible to the Ministry of Local Government and Town Planning, and councillors, although elected every few years, are neither answerable to their electorate on a day-to-day basis nor subject to recall (voting out of office) for unsatisfactory performance. With this extension of the central state to district level, and through the resources available to District Councils, most popular committees, particularly those more recently established, had already become marginalized by 1983. A fragile and evolving system of direct democracy was thus supplanted by representative democracy.

In 1984, the system of local government was further elaborated and extended. As a result of the Prime Minister's directive, decentralized structures were set up 'to facilitate popular participation' in local government. These village development committees (VIDCOs) and ward development committees (WADCOs) were formed 'using popularly elected local leaders to ensure democratic representation in planning development projects for the people'

(Ministry of Community and Cooperative Development 1989). However, these structures are less numerous and more geographically removed from the majority of villagers than were the popular committees which were in attendance at the frequent mass meetings held during 1980 and 1981 at village level.

THE STATE, POPULAR ORGANIZATION, AND HEALTH CARE

If we move from the general sphere of the state to the specific area of health care, how have these developments and contradictions manifested themselves? First of all it is useful to outline those changes enacted by the post-Independence government which have had a positive influence on health and health care.

Post-Independence reforms and their effect on health

Certain economic and social reforms have been instituted which have almost certainly influenced health positively, although some have been eroded, or their progress slowed, since the advent of economic recession and the imposition of structural adjustment measures.

National minimum wages were introduced for all categories of workers in July 1980; they rose substantially until early 1982, whereafter a wage freeze and devaluation of the Zimbabwean dollar resulted in a sharp decline in the real value of wages to pre-July 1980 levels.

Government subsidies on basic foods were removed in 1982 and 1983, resulting in large price increases which have particularly affected low-income households.

Since Independence the government has resettled over 50 000 families, mostly on an individual basis. Adjustment policies resulted in a severe cutback in this programme in 1983, from which it has never regained its momentum.

Zimbabwe's phenomenal post-Independence expansion in school enrolment is likely to contribute significantly to future health status. Total numbers at school grew dramatically: primary enrolments increased from 0.819 million in 1979 to 2.229 million in 1985;

secondary enrolments increased from a mere 79 000 in 1979 to almost half a million in 1985 (Chung 1988).

There has also been a steady improvement in water provision, with over one-third of the communal area population now having access to improved water sources.

Finally, a massive drought relief programme, introduced in 1982, provided a basic food ration to many people between 1982 and 1985, and was undoubtedly critical in mitigating widespread nutritional deterioration (Sanders and Davies 1988).

Transformation of health care services

In line with the new PHC approach, the delivery and management of health care at all levels has been transformed (Loewenson and Sanders 1988; Sanders and Davies 1988). Curative and preventive services have been integrated, and provincial and district health teams established, comprising all the major agencies providing health care, as well as representatives from other sectors and from the relevant local government structures. The hospital doctor is no longer only a curative professional, but is responsible for mobilizing promotive, preventive, curative and rehabilitative services through the health team, as well as training of new cadres and integration with other sectors. Reforms in medical and nursing education and the training of new cadres have also been undertaken.

Other major changes since Independence include:

- Free health care to those earning less than $Z150 per month, who constitute the vast majority of the population. However, since this was enacted in September 1980, increases in workers' minimum wages have disqualified certain groups from receiving this benefit, notwithstanding significant erosion of the real value of these minima.

- A hospital and rural health centre building programme which resulted, by January 1987, in the completion of 274 rural health centres, with a further 49 under construction, and a number of upgraded hospitals.

- The Zimbabwe expanded programme on immunization (ZEPI) which was initiated in 1981. Coverage of children aged 12–23 months increased from 25 per cent in 1982 to 42 per cent in 1984, and to approximately 65 per cent in rural areas in 1986, although since then coverage has stagnated (Ministry of Health 1984*b*).

- A diarrhoeal disease control programme (DDCP) launched in 1982, whose centrepiece has been improved case management through oral rehydration therapy (ORT). Since then, attendance for diarrhoea at health care facilities appears to have decreased, and there has been significant progress in home-based management through ORT.
- An active nutrition programme comprising nutrition education, including breast-feeding promotion, growth-monitoring and nutrition surveillance, and supervision of a national children's supplementary feeding programme (CSFP) and food production programme. The CSFP which operated between 1981 and 1985 post-war period and during the prolonged drought, supplied at its peak a daily energy-rich supplementary meal to over a quarter of a million children in over 8000 rural feeding points. This, and the related drought relief programme, undoubtedly mitigated against widespread nutritional deterioration in this period. However, data suggest that, notwithstanding sharp reductions since Independence in infant and young child mortality, the nutritional status of young children has stagnated, presumably as a result of the deteriorating economic environment.
- Zimbabwe's family planning programme implemented through a parastatal, the Zimbabwe National Family Planning Council (ZNFPC), is reputed to have achieved the highest rate of contraceptive use in sub-Saharan Africa.

Government expenditure and foreign donor aid

These and other programmes required expansion of governmental expenditure. In the first few years following Independence there was rapid expansion of the Ministry of Health (MOH) budget, so that by fiscal year 1981–82 the MOH's actual expenditure had almost doubled in real terms. However, following the downturn in the economy in 1982, and the introduction of economic stabilization measures in 1983, the real growth of 47 per cent in the 1981–82 budget was turned into a real decrease in expenditure of 9.1 per cent in the 1982–83 fiscal year.

The share of preventive services in the MOH budget rose from 7.9 per cent in 1979–80 to 14 per cent in 1985–86, while that of medical care fell from 87.1 per cent to 77.9 per cent. These figures actually understate the shift towards preventive care since some of the costs of such care, especially with respect to immunization, have probably been reduced by the integration of curative and preventive services. This change reflects the impact of the changed philosophy of the MOH after Independence.

The MOH makes major grants to the central hospitals in Harare, to local authorities, missions and voluntary organizations. The central hospitals' share of the MOH budget has been reduced since Independence. The local authorities, missions and voluntary organizations which provide secondary and primary level care received an increased grant between 1980–81 and 1981–82. However, this grant was reduced in the period up to 1985, constraining their ability to perform outreach work.

Thus, government funding of health sector services grew substantially after Independence, but has remained static or grown only slowly since 1981–82. Resources have also been provided by foreign aid donors, whose role has eased some of the constraints faced by government. Although the total amount of aid to the health sector has not been large in comparison with the overall MOH budget, it has been significant in relation to the funding allocated to specific projects. In 1983, 18 per cent of the ZEPI budget came from bilateral and multilateral aid donors. Similarly, the funding for the CSFP came primarily from aid agencies.

Community participation and the nature and role of the VHW

Community participation is one of the hallmarks of the PHC approach adopted enthusiastically in 1978 by all member states of the World Health Organization. It is perhaps community participation and the CHW, or VHW, that particularly distinguish PHC from other strategies previously promoted to improve health and health care provision. Earlier international strategies involved extending health care through the use of 'auxiliaries' or 'paramedics' (King 1966). It has also been argued by some, that the PHC strategy itself could form the basis in the health sector for developing the political strength, organization, and awareness of the popular classes, essential ingredients in the struggle against underdevelopment, and for health (Werner 1981).

However, for the PHC strategy to succeed in the terms suggested above, certain political and economic factors need to obtain. That the thorough implementation of national CHW programmes has so far been relatively dismal, except in countries where radical social transformation has occurred (for example, China), is a salutary reminder of the interlocking of health and politics (Sidel and Sidel 1974; Newell 1975). In those situations where a substantial challenge to the capitalist State by massive and sustained popular mobilizations has occurred, significant improvements in health care and other social service provisions have also often taken place, although the maintenance of these, both in terms of their distribution and especially of their popular involvement and control, relates sensitively to the dynamic of the unfolding class struggle.

Here again, the Zimbabwe case is instructive. Before examining it, however, it is worth recalling the main features, and the political and economic dimensions of VHW schemes within the overall PHC approach.

Some features of VHW schemes

The most important features distinguishing the VHW from the auxiliary are *selection* and *accountability*. In contrast to the auxiliary, the VHWs should be selected by the people they will serve, through a representative body such as a village council or committee, and should be answerable to them, not to the medical profession. In the case of auxiliaries, academic qualifications alone have almost invariably been the criteria used for acceptance into training. The successful experience of both China, and of several small VHW schemes elsewhere, has suggested that compassion and a desire to 'serve the people' are more important qualities (Newell 1975).

As well as being selected by the committees they will serve, VHWs are also meant to be accountable to them. Thus in .Zimbabwe, village committees, or other organs facilitating democratic control by villagers, should retain the responsibility for ongoing liaison with VHWs, constantly bringing to their attention the expressed health and health care needs of the communities they represent, and making known to the VHWs both the satisfaction and dissatisfaction of the people. Ultimately, the authority to dismiss a VHW should rest with the village committee. Equally, the VHWs should be able to transmit through village committees their ideas and perceptions about how committees, or individuals within communities, could or should be involved in health promotion and health care activities.

Technical *supervision and support* of VHWs is usually provided in the first instance by auxiliaries, such as medical assistants and health assistants. Other health care personnel are also required to play a supportive and supervisory role, although they (and indeed all PHC workers) should not be exempt from regular contact with and exposure to popularly elected and representative organs. It is only through such a dialogue that those assuming responsibility for the provision of health services will improve their understanding of the perceived health needs of the vast majority of the people they are attempting to serve, and will thus be in a better position to elaborate more appropriate and appropriable technologies and services. By engaging in such a dialogue, professional health workers will moreover demonstrate their real concern for the people, and their readiness to put their knowledge at the disposal of those whose active participation in successful health promotion and disease control is crucial.

It is important for two reasons that the *work-load* of VHWs is not so great as to prevent them spending a significant fraction of their time in normal productive activities outside the health sector. First, such a division of their time ensures that VHWs do not become 'professionalized' full-time workers, dependent only on their newly-acquired skills for their living, and hence potentially open to the economic attractions of private practice. Second, the continued performance of those production tasks performed by the people whom they are serving helps to ensure that they remain close in perception and experience to their communities. Also, *payment* of the VHW can thus be reduced to subsidization. If the VHWs are to remain responsive to their people then it is important that this subsidy is administered by the community. However, in those countries with poor rural (and urban) communities (and this would apply today in most areas of Zimbabwe) frequently no surplus exists from which a VHW can be subsidized.

Thus it is that most successful VHW schemes either have received substantial funding from a non-governmental (usually foreign) agency, or, after an initial period of reliance on such outside funding, workable health insurance schemes have been devised.

The sustainability of such schemes depends ultimately on how much surplus is produced in the community, and by whom it is controlled. In the preceding period, however, while communities are being afforded the necessary inputs to enable them to regain, and to improve upon, their former productivity, in some instances governments have provided central funding for VHW schemes.*

One of the most important considerations in the development of the VHW was a recognition of the necessity to *extend health care coverage*: the use of health workers based in the community can extend useful, and necessary, health care to many people who would otherwise derive little benefit from the health services. VHWs have great potential to prevent and cure disease and ease suffering through the use of simple technologies. Equipping the VHW with curative skills not only has the effect of providing health care to more people, quickly and more cheaply, but also gives the VHW greater credibility in the eyes of the community.

Moreover, if through education and the use of appropriate technology the VHW is able to equip members of the community with both an understanding of health care and relevant skills, then the medical profession's monopoly of knowledge and expertise is challenged. The power of the doctor, often based on mystification, can in this way be weakened. If certain appropriate health technologies become widely incorporated into health practice, their use can stimulate a critical approach to the expanding range of inappropriately sophisticated, expensive, and mystifying technologies. In this way, conscious self-reliance, that is, self-reliance based on real knowledge, can be fostered.

Perhaps the most important potential of the VHWs is their ability to stimulate within the health sector the *development of the political strength*, *organization and awareness* of the popular classes. David Werner (1981) puts it thus:

> If the village health worker is taught a respectable range of skills, if he is encouraged to think, to take initiative and to keep learning on his own, if his judgment is respected, if his limits are determined by what he knows and can do, if his supervision is supportive and educational, chances are he will work with energy and dedication, will make a major contribution to his community and will win his people's confidence and love. His example

* In Zimbabwe a grant was made from Central Government to District Councils to pay VHWs. This funding was projected to terminate in 1987.

will serve as a role model to his neighbours, that they too can learn new skills and assume new responsibilities, that self-improvement is possible. Thus the village health worker becomes an internal agent-of-change, not only for health care, but for the awakening of his people to their human potential . . . and ultimately to their human rights.

The VHWs' special qualification to play this role as an *agent of social change* derives from two sources, both equally important. First, through the mechanisms of selection and payment, they are more likely to truly represent the people, rather than the medical profession or the State. Second, the VHWs, particularly if working with socially-conscious health workers who can assist in building up an accurate picture of the social roots of ill-health in the area concerned, can endorse ordinary people's beliefs that the sources of their ill-health are rooted in their living and working conditions. For villagers do know that disease is caused by food (or lack of it), bad sanitation and hygiene, poor water supplies, cramped housing, and excessive work.

If VHWs are regarded by the community as their representatives, and respected for their responsiveness and health care capabilities, their effect in confirming the community's understanding of the sources of its ill-health has a powerful potential. This liberating potential is quite the opposite of the negative potential of many health professionals, who transmit the idea that social conditions causing ill-health are natural and unchangeable, and that any solutions rest with the individual.

Problems of VHW schemes

While some local schemes involving VHWs have so far proved very successful, the majority of attempts to institute genuine and effective VHW programmes have failed. There are many reasons for these failures, but some are general and, as will become clear, are manifesting themselves in Zimbabwe now. These problems are indivisible from the general political and economic context, and cannot be specifically adduced to particularities of Ministries of Health.

Economic Problems

In China in the 1960s and 1970s it was acknowledged that in bad agricultural years the funds available for rural health programmes contracted. In those countries with poor rural (and urban) communities, and where production is mostly on an individual basis, frequently no surplus exists from which a VHW can be subsidized. Further, it is often the case that on occasions when a surplus has been created, poor people choose, understandably, to invest in items which they regard as more vital than health care. In fact, they often choose to invest in land or farming implements which undoubtedly contribute more to their health than does health care.

In Mozambique, for example, where a new category of primary health worker, the *agente polivalente*, was developed to work in communal villages, in some villages he/she has to spend most of his/her time producing essential food for the family. Thus, as stated earlier, whether such schemes can be sustained depends in the long term on how much surplus is produced within the community, and who controls it. This, of course, depends on the success or otherwise of the rural development strategy and agricultural policy for the majority, the workers and peasants.

Political problems

Popular, democratic control is a crucial ingredient for the success of a VHW scheme that promotes comprehensive PHC. In communities where most people are poor and often illiterate, the tendency is for the better-off and better-educated to dominate in the decision-making process. This has implications for both the selection and control of the community-based health worker. Indeed, it calls into question the very term 'community', a term which is very freely used, and suggests a homogeneous, conflict-free group of people. This situation almost never exists, particularly in underdeveloped countries. It is not simply that villagers are a different class from professionals. Villagers are also divided among themselves. Communities are stratified by income, social status, and political power.

Hence, it is in situations where the old order and power structures are being contested, or have recently been overthrown, that PHC schemes involving VHWs are more likely to take root. In such conditions, popular participation in decisions, and collective rather than individual self-reliance grows and flourishes.

Eary developments in VHW schemes in Zimbabwe

The evolution of VHW schemes in Zimbabwe since the end of the liberation war provides an illuminating case study of the centrality of politics to the success of such projects and, indeed, to the whole PHC initiative.

Non-government VHW schemes

During the cease-fire period—just before formal Independence—Sister Margaret Nhariwa, a religious sister and health worker at Bondolfi Mission, Masvingo (a province in the south of the country), was involved in developing a VHW programme. She explains its origins:

It's the people who organise themselves and do the choosing; but the way it sprung up in this area was through the party (Zimbabwe African National Union). Not that the party officials came in and said let's do this. But you see during the war there weren't any clinics from here to Mozambique, and the people were sick. So the comrades (guerrillas) took it on themselves to do public health. In this area they were doing public health thoroughly, going visiting homes. When the cease-fire came these people had just taken people on to help them and some of the women were working in the bush hospital treating the guerrillas. Then the people realised that when the guerrillas went they would lose what they had gained in public health. So they approached myself and Father Graf (Father Superior of Bondolfi Mission) and they asked if we could train these people. (Carver 1980; Sanders 1984)

The area was well organized into one political district with 28 branches. Each branch had a committee of sixteen who were popularly elected. Of these sixteen, two were responsible for community health matters. Most of these branch health leaders had had a First Aid Nursing course; some had had one to two years nursing training; a few were qualified nurses and the rest had had no previous health training. Further training commenced at Bondolfi for these 56 branch health leaders in May 1980, and extended over six months. It included both theory and practical work, the latter being done after planning with their committees.

Due to this project's popularity and increasing community demands, the people decided to have an unpaid VHW for every one to three villages, resulting in the selection and training of 293 VHWs, 35 being from other districts.

In the words of Sister Nhariwa, VHWs at Bondolfi were:

selected by the people, voted in. People choose whom they trust, whom they say is kind and whom they say is able and is committed to the community. I think it is the commitment that is looked for much these days, at least in this area. (Carver 1980; Sanders 1984)

It is important to note that selection and control of these workers was at village and branch level with ongoing popular participation. The VHWs were not paid;

When they were trained it was a fighting sort of affair. There were party committees and one doesn't get paid for belonging to a party. So they came in this knowledge that they were doing this for their own people, for the development of their country, and that they had been chosen by the people. (Carver 1980; Sanders 1984)

In describing the training and tasks of the VHWs Sister Nhariwa drew attention to both the comprehensive nature of their work, with its inclusion of promotive, preventive, and curative components, and also the importance accorded to the social causes of ill-health and their solution:

The Village Health Workers are responsible for a village only. They all work to educate mothers and fathers—nutrition, need for wefare clinics, antenatal clinics and public hygiene. They also observe the nutrition state of the people in the village and social problems leading to malnutrition and help solve them locally if possible, or bring them to the party or District if impossible at local level. I would like them to weigh babies—and encourage individual mothers to bring their children to baby clinics who might for fear of after effect—from lack of knowledge—or for shyness because of personal poverty stay away from these necessary public agencies.

They also have to work hand in hand with the Health Assistants in water supply problems and sanitation. The land demonstrators will also come in question. They will have to ask them to teach people who are malnourished because they do not know proper farming. They will see serious illness and send them to Hospital for clinic. They will also see what things can be treated in the home and do it.

But above all, their work is to relate the whole African man with all his beliefs and practices to medicine so that man should not be divided. With the Branch Leaders I have done quite a good bit on the psychology of the African man. They of course knew more than I so they discussed and helped each other with what I thought was a sound beginning. Their course takes two weeks at the start. Then they come back once every month for a report back and some lectures for six months. We will then have a kind of graduation ceremony. I will go round seeing their work and co-ordinating it.

I teach mostly on a discussion basis. In the discussions come up the social problems from the students. I give them a few questions which relate to social problems and social causes of poor health and that way the whole section on social problems is thrashed out and then they discuss possible solutions to the problems.

This syllabus is of course in need of correction. I have adapted it for village health workers in the rural areas. These people have become, as I experienced whilst teaching them, very much aware of their needs and their social problems. And they are also convinced they have a big part to play in the solving of these health problems. Of course in the first lesson I give them the structure of health as it stands in our country.

Before we have solved the social problems it is very difficult to solve some of the health problems in Zimbabwe. Therefore the need to make people aware of the social problems relating to health. (Sanders 1980)

With remarkable foresight, Sister Margaret pinpointed the critical economic factor in this project's future success:

I do appreciate these people who have voluntarily offered to have a course—though chosen by the masses—so as to work for the development of others for no pay. It is a pity they have no income support in this. Because even if they are so eager as they are today, their own personal needs will one day draw them back. They have given me an example which is moving. (Sanders 1980)

From this project sprang up a Development Committee, organized by the people themselves.

Its aim is to co-ordinate the work done by VHWs in different areas, and organise other development projects that are not directly involved with health . . . The formation of the Development Committee has strengthened the health projects and intensified these projects, making the people more determined than ever. (Carver 1980; Sanders 1984)

Government VHW programmes

Soon after Independence, the Government stated that essential basic health services would be made accessible to the majority of the population, especially in the neglected rural areas—and underlined its commitment to the PHC approach.

One of the first few programmes to be launched was the National Village Health Worker Programme. This programme, although centrally planned and initiated, was strikingly similar in many respects to the Bondolfi project. Ministry of Health documents describe the context as well as the objectives and establishment of the VHW scheme:

In mapping out the course for the extension of health services to our rural populations therefore, we have found it necessary to move towards the strategy which emphasises the setting up of many smaller and evenly distributed low cost units countrywide i.e. the health centres. These health centres will be manned by Medical and Health Assistants who will work in conjunction with, as well as supervise, the frontline grassroots workers—*The Village Health Workers*.

The Village Health Worker is a man, or woman, who is selected by his/her community to promote health education and motivate the community members in the promotion of health education activities. Village Health Workers receive a 12 week training course offered by the Ministry of Health, during which they learn about personal and home hygiene, advantages of proper sanitation, nutrition, preventative measures, first aid and management of minor and common ailments such as childhood gastroenteritis and common skin infections.

It is the Ministry's goal that eventually each community will have its own Village Health Worker.

The National objectives to the Village Health Worker Scheme are:

1. To ensure that each community has a grassroot worker chosen by its members to promote health education in that community, thereby making basic health care accessible to all.

2. To give the community the opportunity to participate actively in the promotion of its own health.

3. To ensure that each community is in a position to mobilise local resources and technical assistance necessary for the provision of potable water supplies and proper sanitation.

In order to achieve these objectives the primary health care plan was developed and at the primary level it included:

1. Increasing and expanding the rural health centres as these would provide the necessary back-up support needed by the Village Health Workers.
2. Orienting health workers to Primary Health Care especially those working in rural and preventive services.
3. Orienting the communities to Primary Health Care, its objectives and proposed strategies for implementation.
4. Establishing the training programme of Village Health Workers nationally. (Ministry of Health)

Workshops were held at provincial level both to orient health staff to PHC and to appraise local government staff, including District

Councillors, of PHC and the role and functions of VHWs. Written guide-lines were issued to Councillors concerning both VHW selection, training, function, and accountability, as well as the role of Councillors, Health Committees, and the Community in the VHW programme.

The criteria upon which VHWs were to be selected (Ministry of Health 1982) were listed thus:

1.1 Need for stability. The prospective candidate must be a permanent resident in the community.

1.2 Need for a candidate who is of the same cultural/socio-economic/tribal background as the community one is serving.

1.3 Must be a lively and good community motivator. Primarily the role of the Village Health Worker is promoting health and preventing of diseases.

1.4 Must be a person respected, and accepted by the community. One whom the community trusts, and one who can inspire confidence in the community.

1.5 Must be able to identify with the masses of the community and not be seen as an alien whose intentions may be suspect.

1.6 Knowledge of basic reading, writing, as well as keeping of simple records is essential. Knowledge of English should not be taken as a criteria. We should see literacy as being related to any vernacular language, while bearing in mind that English is a foreign language, not spoken conversantly by a large section of our community, notably those in the rural areas.

The role of councillors, the health committee, and the community were also spelt out:

Role of Councillors:

1. Inform and educate community about selection of Village Health Workers and what community should expect from VHWs.
2. Encourage community participation and support of the activities of VHWs.
3. Funds to pay VHWs will be given to the Councillors.
4. Help to monitor activities of Health Committee and Village Health Workers.

When you go back you need to organise meetings in your wards—educate the people. (Trainers help). Councillors do not choose VHW but organise to facilitate selection.

Role of Health Committee:

1. There must be one on each village level. Together with VHW they meet and determine what the health needs of the community are and how the VHW can help them.
2. They also must be supportive and attend meetings when called by VHW.
3. Review progress related to health and the activities of the VHW.
4. Information provided by Health Committee and VHW will be used for in-service (training) after the first three months of practice.

Role of Community:

1. Select the Village Health Worker.
2. Be active in carrying out projects or activities initiated by VHWs.
3. Appreciate that even though he/she works part-time, he/she may work for many hours on some occasions and should therefore assist him or her with her work such as harvesting, mowing, ploughing.

The Councillors are the people who have to make the community accept this programme as *their* programme. They have to teach the people what PHC means, why the Government has chosen it and also encourage the community to be self-reliant.

The funds which the Ministry of Health is making available to pay the VHWs will be given to the Councils, who will in turn pay the VHW, and if the VHW has to be away for some time out of his/her community, he/she should make the Council aware of this. The *Health Committee* is responsible for the support of the VHW. Together they should call the village meetings to discuss health matters with the community. They will review with the VHW health problems and the health activities which should be priority.

The community selects, the whole community should support the VHW in as many ways as is possible, for instance even though we say the VHW works part time, we know that in practice there may be days or seasons when she puts in long hours in giving assistance, for example in the summer when there is a lot of diarrhoea, etc. The community should therefore assist her with ploughing her fields, harvesting, hoeing, etc.

The community should further be active in the projects of self sufficiency and self reliance activities which the VHWs will be promoting, for example if the community is asked to participate in digging a well or digging pit latrines, etc.

And of course, the community should be interested in all activities of health, come to meetings when they are called to discuss health matters, because it is only if the community is interested that the VHWs scheme will be successful.

Furthermore, the Government is hopeful that after one–two years the communities will begin to take some of the responsibility to pay all or part of the salary of the VHWs, because about eleven thousand to twelve thousand VHWs are needed to cover the whole country, and at that point it will be difficult for the Government to pay them all. (Ministry of Health 1982)

In May 1981, senior community health nurses, two from each province, underwent a short workshop to prepare them to function as tutors of the trainers of VHWs. In June–July 1981, the course for trainers of VHWs commenced in the five provincial training centres. Two trainers (medical and health assistants) from each of the 55 districts attended these 12-week courses. In October–November 1981, the training of 344 VHWs started in the 55 districts. Most districts had six VHWs with a few having 7–10 trainees. After their 12-week course, VHWs returned to their villages and each was to be visited by a trainer and a tutor, ongoing technical support being provided by the PHC workers (medical assistants and health assistants) based at the local health centre.

Between 1982 and 1987, 900–1000 VHWs were trained annually, so that by early 1987 about 7000 had been trained out of a final target of 15 000 (Ministry of Health, personal communication).

Although each VHW was ultimately to be responsible for 50–100 households, or 500–1000 people (Ministry of Health 1983*b*), the small number of VHWs present in each district, particularly in the early years of the programme, meant that much larger numbers of people, and far greater distances needed to be covered by each VHW. Many reports indicate that this has rendered them more full-time than part-time in their activities, contributing to the danger of their potential 'professionalization'.

Community participation in Zimbabwe's national VHW programme

The Government White Paper, 'Planning for Equity in Health' outlined the government's 'health policy consistent with the economic policy which seeks to establish a socialist, egalitarian and democratic society in Zimbabwe' (Ministry of Health 1984*a*). In this document the essence of the relationship between the VHWs and their community is stressed:

It should be emphasised that these workers are not extensions of the government health service. They should not so much provide health care for the village, as be an expression of the village's collective commitment to promote their own health; in this process the VHW provides technical guidance. It will be a concern of the government to ensure that community health involvement does not become an empty watchword, and the VHW does not degenerate simply into a first-aid worker, as has happened in so many other countries.

Village health workers will become the key link between the organised village community and the local health service. They are selected by their own communities at mass meetings convened by the village and branch committees, and in this process the chief criteria should be their political commitment to serve the village and, if at all possible, basic literacy. Most VHWs will be peasants, who, at least in the beginning, will work part-time on health. Eventually it will be the responsibility of the communities to provide for the VHWs subsistence needs, but at present the villages are very poor, and in this situation the VHWs will be given an allowance by the District Council out of a grant provided by the Ministry of Health. The VHWs remain responsible, however, to their communities represented by the village and branch committees.

The centrality of popular democratic control to the effective functioning of the reformed health service is made explicit in the White Paper:

This principle of mutual respect and dialogue is at the heart of the new relationship to be created between the health service and the community. Both sides will benefit. The people will feel the health units and activities are 'theirs', and will utilise and participate in them as such. The health workers will receive a boost to their morale and motivation, their activities, being responsive to the local situation, will be more effective and more efficient in the use of resources.

This new relationship should not be limited to the periphery of the health system, but should permeate all levels of the service, up to the central hospitals. In the past, many of the country's health personnel, notably the professionals, have suffered from an occupational disease, that of paternalism and delusions of 'knowing all'. An active popular involvement in health affairs should help these workers to overcome their superiority complexes, be they in relation to the public in general, to black Zimbabweans in particular, or to more junior members of the health service.

Just as the public should have representation on health services structures, and have channels through which to lodge complaints in the event of bad treatment, so junior health staff should have the opportunity to participate in discussions and decision-making. These are two facets of the same process, that of debureaucratisation and democratisation of the health service, in which hierarchical relationships will be two-way, and there will be much stronger feedback communications from the base upwards. This is a political question which must have repercussions in the whole health sector. (Ministry of Health 1984*a*)

In the light of the above challenging and progressive policy statements, and of the early, popularly-based Bondolfi VHW initiative, what has been the experience of community participation in Zimbabwe's National VHW Programme?

1982 evaluation

A number of formal evaluations, both national and local, of the Government programme have been performed since its inception. While these all assessed a wide range of areas, the most revealing findings relate to the political, rather than the technical, aspects of this scheme. The first evaluation was conducted in early 1982, after the first batch of VHWs had been in the field for a period of 8–10 weeks. A total of 66 VHWs and 121 community members were interviewed. Even at this early stage it emerged that:

although 97 per cent of the VHWs said they had been selected by members of the community, only 35 per cent of the community members said they had been involved in the selection. (Ministry of Health 1982)

That Councillors are indeed only intermittently in communication with villagers was revealed by the finding that, only 31 per cent of community members had first learned about the VHW project from the Councillors, with 22 per cent and 14 per cent having heard of it from clinic staff and friends or neighbours respectively (Ministry of Health 1982). Although 80 per cent of the community members interviewed had heard about the VHW project, and 45 per cent had either had contact with, or participated in an activity organized by the VHW, 49 per cent had not heard of anything taking place in their village that involved the VHW. The evaluation report suggested this low percentage was a result of both the fact that the VHWs had only been in the field for eight weeks, and that they also had very large areas to cover.

Only 30 per cent of the VHWs reported receiving help with their own daily chores from the community members. When the VHWs were asked what problems they had in undertaking their work, 32 per cent said the area they had to cover was too big, 17 per cent said lack of medicines, and 14 per cent indicated that poor response from the community had been a major problem (Ministry of Health 1982).

Among the recommendations made in the evaluation report were, first, that community leaders should be guided in stressing to the community the importance of helping the VHW, and second, that communities should be enlightened:

> on the voluntary community based aspect of the VHW's work to facilitate her acceptance as a community member giving service rather than a fully employed civil servant. (Ministry of Health 1982)

1983 evaluation

The evaluation performed in 1983, while concerned with the overall impact of the activities of VHWs throughout the country (Ministry of Health 1983*b*), investigated certain aspects of 'community participation' in this scheme. Surprisingly, only 37 per cent of the 470 community members interviewed indicated that they knew who paid the VHWs. Of this 37 per cent, 54 per cent (that is, approximately 20 per cent of the total) believed the VHWs to be paid by the District Councils. The evauation report took this to indicate that:

> to a large extent the community sees the VHW as one of the health workers who is mainly accountable to the government or its officials and minimally accountable to the community. It should be noted that many health workers working at the rural council clinics are paid through district councils and many community members seem to place the VHW in the same category. (Ministry of Health 1983*b*)

Of the 95 VHWs interviewed, although 91 per cent claimed to 'be supported' by their communities, it was only in isolated cases that the community support included assisting the VHW with her own work at home or in the fields (Ministry of Health 1983*b*). 65 per cent of VHWs claimed to be morally and practically supported by Councillors, 37 per cent by their trainers, 55 per cent by local health assistants, and 44 per cent by the other health workers. Only 26 per cent of the VHWs noted the presence of health committees (sub-committees of the local community development committees) in their areas, and of these 78 per cent (that is only 20 per cent of the total number) had good communications with these community bodies (Ministry of Health 1983*b*).

Finally, 55 per cent of community members interviewed in 1983 indicated that the VHWs' allowance was insufficient to meet their needs. This prompted a recommendation by the evaluators that 'ways in which communities could be motivated to give tangible support to the VHW be investigated' (Ministry of Health 1983*b*).

There was, however, no recommendation issued concerning health committees, or other structures to facilitate popular involvement in health, notwithstanding the above finding and the recommendation made in the 1982 evaluation report concerning 'the voluntary/community–based aspect of the VHW's work'.

1984 PHC Review

In 1984, a comprehensive national PHC Review was performed, the first part 'concentrating on the community-based element which includes the VHWs and their support system' (Ministry of Health 1984*c*). This evaluation involved interviews with health staff and agencies—government and non-government—at all levels of the health sector, including central and community levels, as well as with VHWs, traditional midwives, families and local leaders.

While presented in the most subtle terms the results of the review at a central level were, none the less, revealing:

> The overall impression, resulting from the 24 interviews of high level staff in Harare, was that there was a commitment to the PHC approach by all concerned.
>
> Ministries realised the need for decentralization and more intersectoral co-ordination, and the need for extending coverage with services. At the central Ministry Headquarters, the elements of community participation, the need for effective communication with and sensitization of communities and the problems of support of village health workers may seem remote. It is perhaps more expedient to have initially central control and uniformity

of services for the whole country than to have a system that responds to variable locally expressed interests and wants. However, now with decentralization increased community participation will become more prominent as an essential aspect of programmes. The International Aid Agencies, not so involved in country wide implementation, however, put an emphasis on community involvement and communication . . .

. . . As discussions are going on at policy-making level on the future of the VHW programme, it can be assumed that the aspect of remuneration is also being dealt with. It is crucial and tied up with community involvement and with the possibility of ultimate coverage of all the communities in the country. (Ministry of Health 1984*c*)

At provincial level it was noted that:

The steps already taken to facilitate PHC are on the whole steps that need to be taken even further. Few details of the training workshops required in future were given by most provinces: they would presumably be linked to the steps still required. These are motivation of health committees, arousing community awareness . . . intersectoral co-ordination . . . Further decentralization requires bold steps . . . Intersectoral co-ordination at provincial level did not appear to be strong . . . Education and Community Development and Women's Affairs both having staff down to community level would appear to be the most useful allies, and yet were hardly mentioned. (Ministry of Health 1984*c*)

At district level it was observed that:

The district team members are however the ones showing the greatest changes in their routines to facilitate PHC and in line with decentralization. (Ministry of Health 1984*c*)

None the less, it was still noted:

The district team interviewed were remarkable for the high proportion of less experienced officers acting in the absence of the incumbent of the position. This implies a need for orientation of all trained staff towards PHC, and not only the 4 people who are often transferred or absent. This absence of orientation was probably the reason for the lack of emphasis on mobilization and sensitization of communities and the establishment of co-ordinated intersectoral activities. (Ministry of Health 1984*c*)

That the earlier mentioned obsession with geographical equality in the development of the national VHW scheme had led to a problem of inadequate coverage of communities is reflected in the following comment:

This one district also brings into clear focus the problem of producing enough VHWs to ensure that they are assigned to a community rather than a ward (6 villages with an estimated population of 6000 people). (Ministry of Health 1984*c*)

This is reinforced later in the review, when it was recognized that the low density of VHWs has led to their becoming virtually full-time workers, rendering them closer in experience to their professional mentors than to their communities:

The present coverage of homes by a single VHW means that they are hardly village health workers and unable to function as such—they take on the role of an assistant to the HA, and concentrate on spreading one or two ideas, e.g. pot racks. If the VHW had a real community to deal with, then perhaps the mother and children would come into focus and an emphasis on MCH, growth charts, immunization would be possible. (Ministry of Health 1984*c*)

The findings at health centre level—the level from which VHWs are supervised--were revealing:

Both cadres (Medical Assistants and Health Assistants) conceived of PHC as the provision of services such as sanitation, water, MCH (maternal and child health) and immunization. There was little emphasis on community involvement and motivation (possibly more emphasis by HA), and integration and co-ordination with other sectors was hardly considered. The features of PHC which distinguish it from all that went before are total coverage, community participation and intersectoral co-ordination, and these must be stressed more in future in-service training. The basis to achieve them, e.g. epidemiology, communication and improved management need more emphasis also.

The time spent on VHWs by MA was small, whereas HA spent considerable time with them. More team work between the two is needed, and also the MA needs to get out to group meetings more if the Health Centre is to become truly community oriented. A Health Centre with community leaders on its committee or team was not prominent. ((Ministry of Health 1984*c*)

In common with the findings in the 1982 evaluation it was observed:

The Village Health Workers interviewed were mostly women and their age, marital status, parity, being born in the area and education were all in keeping with good selection, which also seemed to be borne out by the almost universal claim to have been selected by the people at a public gathering. However, comments by health staff and community members implied a certain element of selection by councillors in the beginning of the programme. One reported case of community dissatisfaction with a VHW and his defection was directly related to lack of selection based on community consensus. This problem is overcome by lengthier preparation and sensitization of communities. ((Ministry of Health 1984*c*)

Later, the review observes:

VHWs do work with other extension workers, mostly Health Assistants, home economics demonstrators and agricultural assistants. This is excellent and in future can perhaps be reinforced by meetings of the Village Development (Health) Committees, which appear to be starting to function, and on which many VHWs serve. These committees have an important role to play in support of VHW and actually need training in this role. (Ministry of Health 1984*c*)

It is illuminating of the government's bureaucratic approach to community development' to note that, in 1984, centrally initiated Village Development Committees were being identified as important supportive structures for this programme, whereas those 'spontaneously' created in 1980 in the Bondolfi scheme were neither supported, nor was their replication in other geographical areas encouraged by the government.

In summary the reviewers highlight the centralized and inflexible nature of this government programme:

This review of the village health worker programme has shown that it has been established in a uniform way throughout all provinces of Zimbabwe. Training, continuing education and supervision are also taking place according to a pattern set by the headquarters.

Although the structures are now in place (decentralization with district and village committees) they are not yet functioning with optimum effect, nor is there great emphasis on the strategies of community participation and multi-sectoral involvement for health. As a consequence of the delayed development of these aspects, there is as yet little evidence of locally planned area specific programmes.

The pattern of training and the system of remuneration of the VHWs do not appear to stimulate community involvement in health care. A less didactic form of training with more emphasis on communication and social processes, and more involvement of village committees, political channels, and other sectors such as Education and Community Development and

Women's affairs should lead to great community participation'. (Ministry of Health 1984*c*)

In response to the findings of this review a number of recommendations were made concerning among other areas, 'community participation in the VHW programme'. A selection of these follows (Ministry of Health 1984*c*):

- Headquarters staff (of all Ministries concerned with health development) together with key International Agencies and NGO leadership should have periodic 'continuing education' workshops on PHC, emphasizing such aspects as community involvement and communication for development.
- A task force should be constituted to look into remuneration of VHWs, and on the numbers to be trained and size of their community to be covered.
- The provincial co-ordinator of trainers needs an assistant with training in preparation of training material and community participation approaches.
- The next round of training workshops at provincial level should cover motivation of health committees, community sensitization, modification of training programmes, increased emphasis on MCH, intersectoral co-ordination, supervision of VHWs.
- Districts should organise a joint workshop for Health Centre area health assistants and other extension workers. It should cover supervision of VHW and TM (traditional midwife), community participation, co-ordination between sectors, communication and information processing.
- VHW training should put more emphasis on communication and social processes.
- Selection of VHW requires community meetings to gain consensus on method of selection and orientation in relation to job description.
- School teachers, political leaders and councillors should be given training in PHC and the role of VHWs..

It is somewhat ironic, given the scant attention, support and publicity given to the Bondolfi scheme by the Government, that the final recommendation of this review states:

Individual NGO successful innovation and community approaches should be more widely known in a district so that they can be replicated. ((Ministry of Community Cooperative Development, undated)

Recent developments

Demise of the Bondolfi programme

It was earlier noted that the nascent dual power situation in rural Zimbabwe was critically affected, and the embryonic popular state weakened, by the expansion of the centralized state and its extension through new local government bodies. The Bondolfi VHW scheme which arose out of, and was organically linked to, the popular mobilization, suffered a similar fate. In the district of Masvingo, where the Bondolfi scheme was based, the commencement of the national progamme proved problematic. Of the almost 300 Bondolfi VHWs, 10 were taken into the government programme and trained. Because of their much lower concentration in the population in this national programme they had to cover much larger areas than the Bondolfi women: in effect most became full-time workers.

Further, the payment received by them from the District Council, although termed 'an allowance', was inevitably viewed by their former colleagues as a salary. In the words of an organizer of the Bondolfi VHW scheme:

When the government scheme started and some were paid 33 dollars a month, others stopped working because they were not being paid. (Carver 1980; Sanders 1984)

Although there are other reasons, this factor was undoubtedly significant in the slow demise of the Bondolfi programme. By mid-1984 only about 100 VHWs were still working, and recent information suggests that only a small number of the original workers continue to function. The decline in this project and demoralization among its workers is unfortunate. It reflects a process of centralization, bureaucratization, and devaluation of popular initiative, and, signifies a reversal from a situation where popular involvement in political, social and economic activities was fairly widespread, to one where people's participation is generally mediated through 'representative', but distant, bodies such as District Councils and, more recently, Ward Committees and Village Committees.

Weaknesses of government programmes

Ever since the first programme evaluation it has emerged clearly that their communities have frequently regarded the government VHWs as selected by and accountable to government officials. In 1984, the national organizer of the government programme was disarmingly frank when asked about its weaknesses:

> Well, some people leave because they are not satisfied. There is some nepotism, councillors choose their wives, and friends, but these say 'I can make more than $30 a month selling a box of tomatoes, so I'm resigning'. We are not present when they are chosen and it will take time to see that they root out nepotism. Also there is administrative competition. [The Ministry of] Women's Affairs think that since most VHWs are women, they should be under them, but we have the expertise, and they don't. Other Ministries have their interest too. (Quoted in Sanders 1984.)

The politically problematic nature of 'community participation' in VHW schemes—and indeed in PHC in general—has already been referred to. The relative presence or absence of accountability of VHWs to their 'communities' reflects the extent and depth of the democratic process. Since about 1982, effective popular involvement in the social and political process in general, and in the VHW programme in particular, has declined inversely in relation to bureaucratization and nepotism. The latter's persistence is illustrated in a 1988 report from a district in eastern Zimbabwe, where popular mobilization and self-organization were well-developed in the early post-Independence period:

> . . . the people here are highly politicized and know their rights. They also have the resolve, and the will, to spontaneously participate in activities affecting their lives. Unfortunately, the rural elite usually frustrate this political activity. For example some district councillors were suppressing community views, choosing their wives or relatives to village health worker posts. Some health workers were only working with 'well to do, motivated' families who could make projects successful. As a result many projects benefited the well to do, while the poor and disadvantaged became poorer and more disadvantaged. However the communities have been able to vote out some of the corrupt officials although a lot more needs to be done. (Tumwine 1988)

It is evident then that, notwithstanding the recognition in successive evaluations of the related problems of professionalization of VHWs, nepotism in their selection and bureaucratization and centralization of the programme, these deficiencies appear to have persisted. Although the 1984 PHC Review made explicit and specific recommendations for corrective action, it is not clear how many of the suggestions were implemented: the author is unaware of any significant initiatives along the lines suggested.

However, although a piecemeal approach to these defects in the VHW programme, which are essentially reflections of fundamental political problems, would have ameliorated some of the problems, it would probably not have succeeded without an accompanying more generalized assault on the power of those groups who have come to dominate political structures at both local and central levels. The most potent and reliable constraint on nepotism, bureaucratization, and anti-democratic practices is the encouragement and extension of popular democratic control, the beginnings of which were visible in the wake of the liberation struggle.

The new cadre of Village Community Worker

More recent developments have crystallized certain of the above negative tendencies evident in earlier years. Bureaucratic rivalry between the Ministry of Health and the Ministry of Community Cooperative Development and Women's Affairs (MCCDWA) has finally been resolved with the signing, by the two Ministries on 2 February 1987, of an agreement transferring responsibility for this programme to the MCCDWA.

The Village Community Worker (VCW) as this new cadre is termed, is a village-based, multi-purpose worker with wide-ranging responsibilities, including many of the former VHW's tasks. VCWs have been formed by amalgamation of the former VHWs with the former Home Economics Demonstrators (operatives of the MCCDWA), as well as recruitment of new VCWs.

The job description for the VCW, as shown below has reasonably been criticized for being too broad and demanding (Ministry of Community Cooperative Development 1988):

1. Work with the Village Development Committee, in identifying and evaluating village problems relating to health, agriculture,

community education, child spacing, pre-schools, women's issues, and assist with community action where necessary.

2. Liaise with the village person responsible for adult literacy, pre-schools, and promotion of youth and women's activities.
3. Encourage the formation of interest groups such as savings clubs, women's clubs, and support their uniform-making, vegetable gardens, and so on.
4. To make personal visits to homes and motivate mothers for antenatal and post-natal care, and also to mobilize and teach communities about basic hygiene measures, water and sanitation, general health education, treat minor illnesses, refer people to clinics, and offer advice on other services that may be required.
5. Mobilize communal farmers for agricultural and conservation issues.
6. Keep a register of chronically ill patients within the village.
7. Report to the nearest Health Centre monthly to submit information on number of births and deaths in the village.
8. Establish and maintain a dialogue with traditional midwives.
9. Help families identify and cope with physically or mentally handicapped people for rehabilitation and for early referral and treatment.
10. Mobilize communities to form co-operative movements through income generating projects.

The process of implementing the VCW programme was similar to that for the VHW, with the provincial and district training teams being developed in 1988, and the training of VCWs then commencing.

The tendency towards professionalization observed in the VHW programme has been further strengthened by a number of factors. The most important of these are the criteria for consideration as a VCW laid down by the MCCDWA. Candidates require at least seven years of primary education, should be under 45 years of age and healthy (Shearly and Woelk, personal communication).

In contrast to VHWs, VCWs have promotional prospects. Promotion of VCWs to Ward Community Co-ordinators, who are salaried employees of the MCCDWA, is possible for 'hard working cadres' (Ministry of Community Cooperative Development 1988), although one District Medical Officer implies that academic attainment is also a factor:

> The Village Community Workers (VCWs) as the new cadres are now called, are disillusioned about the proposed career structure where academic achievement is the most important criterion for promotion.
>
> Yet some of the very good VCWs elected by their communities have no hope of promotion as they are too old to obtain their grade seven, or ZJC, let alone 'O' levels. (Tumwine 1988)

It has also been suggested that the present VCW should be 'upgraded . . . to full-time worker status'. (Ministry of Community Cooperative Development 1988)

It is clear from the above that there is a definite blurring of the difference in status between this cadre and a full-time civil servant, which is so fundamental to the conception of the VHW.

Relationship of VCWs to the community

This process of metamorphosis of a community representative into a civil servant—best exemplified by the Bondolfi VHW—has been enhanced by an apparent confusion on the part of government officials in their understanding of the relationship of the VCW to the community. This lack of clarity has had implications for the selection and accountability of the cadre. Government documents refer to problems in the relationship between VHWs and VIDCOs, implying that it is these community representative bodies which have an incorrect perception of the nature of the VCW. In an early document it was stated:

> A clear distinction should be made between VIDCOs and Village Community Worker responsibilities, of which the former need to be educated on the role and responsibility of the latter. Presently there are signs of power struggle between these. (Ministry of Community Cooperative Development 1988)

Similarly, more than a year later, at the MCCDWA's National Consultative Workshop for Provincial Training Teams, it was observed:

> The training of Village Community Workers resulted in the existence of a strained relationship between them and VIDCOs. The latter felt their

positions were threatened. Definitely the training the cadres received would make them very influential, and the relationship was worsened by the fact that the Village Community Workers were getting an allowance. (Ministry of Community Cooperative Development 1989)

There is none the less still a recognition by Ministry workers of the central importance of a sound community base for the successful functioning of the VCW scheme:

The Village Community Workers can only operate smoothly where there are well established development structures at village level. There is need to establish and strengthen the operations of WADCOs and VIDCOs. (Ministry of Community Cooperative Development 1989)

However, it appears that genuine confusion persists among senior MCCDWA officials as to the direction of accountability of the VCW. It is suggested by the following ruminating discussion at the National Consultative Workshop that a clear distinction between political accountability (to the 'community') and technical responsibility (to the MCCDWA) is not being made:

This cadre who is supposed to supervise the Village Community Workers needs skills on type of supervision to be given. This needs careful thought since the programme is a little tricky and confusing to many. According to the PM's (Prime Minister's) directive the Village Community Worker is accountable to the community which selected him/her, and reports to VIDCO chairperson her day to day activities. Somehow, it is felt somebody with authority to monitor work output should be placed above this cadre. Does this mean direct control or not? Other Ministries want to monitor to what extent the Village Community Worker is promoting their activities, and need to do this closely with the Ward Community Co-ordinator. It is with this confusion in mind that it was felt there is a need to train Ward Community Co-ordinators on what their role in supervising the Village Workers would be. (Ministry of Community Cooperative Development 1989)

Clearly, however, in certain peripheral settings where implementation of the VCW scheme is occurring, the status of the VCW is not even in doubt, and is certainly not to be allowed to interfere with the priorities of the local bureaucracy. This is starkly illustrated by the following observation made by a Medical Officer in Nyanga District close to the country's eastern border:

Of particular concern to the health service must be the directive given to our local VHWs at a recent meeting, when they were addressed by a senior administrative officer of the Ministry of Community Development, who told them that they were now employees of a ministry *other than* the Ministry of Health and, henceforth, such activities as attending ZEPI (Zimbabwe Expanded Programme on Immunization) points might lead to their dismissal! (Smyly 1988)

Here again bureaucratic control and bureaucratic rivalry manifest as strong and negative factors of a government programme.

Another unfortunate effect of the changeover from the VHW to the VCW programme, is that the amalgamation of the Ministry of Health programme with that of the MCCDWA has caused a situation where:

some villages already have more Village Community Workers than are needed and withdrawing some will create problems. (Ministry of Community Cooperative Development 1988)

The final outcome of the rivalry between these two Ministries which have competed for 'control' of this programme is, it seems, a situation where communities are being, indirectly and no doubt unintentionally, victimized. A study performed by a District Nursing Officer in Chimanimani District in Eastern Zimbabwe in 1988 found, that a high percentage of VCWs were no longer involved in health activities, that they were overworked and the 'majority expressed lack of co-ordination between the Ministries of Health and Community Co-operative Development and Women's Affairs'. (Shearly 1988)

An equally disturbing finding was that:

The health supervisors themselves had stopped to give the VCWs support that they used to hence their complete disassociation with the Rural Health Centre staff. This response was supported by the majority of the health staff who said they thought these cadres were no longer their responsibility, since they had been transferred to another ministry. (Shearly 1988)

Many nurses who were interviewed stated that they were not happy to issue VCWs with drugs, as they had lost touch with them and were no longer getting written reports from the VCWs enabling them to monitor drug usage. This was confirmed by the MCCDWA supervisors, who informed the health centre staff that they could get such information from interministerial reports lodged with the Community Development supervisors! (Shearly 1988). One disturbing result of this has been an increase in the number of patients defaulting in their drug treatment (Shearly 1988).

CONCLUSION

In Zimbabwe there have been major reforms in the health sector since Independence, many as a result of decisions taken at central level, and some from the actions at a more peripheral level of individuals and groups, both in government employment and outside it. These progressive reforms are ultimately a reflection of the fact that a state which has not yet consolidated itself following a major shift in power—such as the Zimbabwean state in 1980–82—is sometimes susceptible to pressure from the popular classes. However, progressive moves by states as well as those by individuals are subject to definite limits. These are imposed by the ebb in the class struggle, sometimes initiated and aggravated by conscious policies of popular demobilization, and by the regional and international political context.

The case study of VHWs discussed above is one illustration of the dynamic and complex relationship between, and within, the state and the popular classes. Clearly this experience was one which existed in a complex set of specific conditions. However, it was not an isolated phenomenon; similar centralization and bureaucratization has affected *inter alia* the co-operative movement and trade union movement (Ministry of Community Cooperative Development 1989).

The possibility of true 'community participation', or to be more precise, of democratization within the health sector, is inseparable from the process of democratization within all institutions of society. This process is a direct reflection of the level and tempo of the class struggle. Democratic control by the popular classes is the central core of the PHC strategy, for it is, and will be, the mechanism through which health and health care resources will be more equitably allocated and more appropriate to the majority's needs.

8

The limits of participation in health: *brigadista* programmes in Nicaragua

EDWARD COYLE, GEORGE DAVEY SMITH AND PETER SANDIFORD

INTRODUCTION

The development of health services in Nicaragua following the popular revolution in 1979 has particular international relevance, since this period coincides with the programme for primary health care (PHC) launched by the World Health Organization and UNICEF at the Alma-Ata Conference (WHO 1978*a*). PHC was an essential component of the WHO programme for 'Health for All by the Year 2000'. For developing countries community health workers (CHWs) were seen to be 'the most realistic solution for attaining total population coverage with essential health services'. The origin of CHWs from the communities they served, and the continuous participation of the community in the quest for health, were advanced as key elements in this strategy.

The PHC programme was launched with enormous enthusiasm. However, in the period following Alma-Ata, disillusion set in when it became apparent that CHWs had become 'just another pair of hands' in many settings (Walt 1990). Attempts to account for why PHC failed to function as intended have focused upon the lack of the political support required to facilitate the necessary structural change (Heggenhougen 1987). The required political support would need to deal with the groups against whose interests PHC would run. Often, of course, the existing governments constituted one such interest group. The community involvement, engendered by participatory health care strategies, could be viewed as being threatening to current governments, in that the desire for self-determination could spread and encompass demands for broader involvement in the social process (Werner 1981). Inadequate or antagonistic political action has thus been seen as a key factor in the contribution of disappointing outcomes in many PHC and CHW programmes (Ugalde 1985).

In this regard, examination of the Nicaraguan example is instructive, since the post-revolutionary government had a vigorous commitment to PHC, which has been recognized by the regional office of the WHO for the Americas. This commitment allows the Nicaraguan experience to be viewed as a demonstration of the possibilities and limitations of the PHC strategy, given appropriate political support. This chapter will examine the PHC programme within Nicaragua, in regard to the broader health, social, and political activities from which it cannot be analytically separated. Since the community health volunteers (usually known as *brigadistas*) have had particular symbolic and actual importance within Nicaragua's PHC strategy, they will be the main focus of the discussion.

BACKGROUND

In 1979, Nicaragua's Gross National Product was averaged at $800 for each of its estimated 2.7 million inhabitants (Inter-American Development Bank 1979). Its population structure was that of a developing country in demographic transition, with a median age of 19 years (Fewer 1982). The fertility rate was high, estimated in 1975 at 6.5 per thousand per year. Since 1979 the population has grown to an estimated 3.5 million (INEC-CELADE, Nicaragua 1983).

Nicaragua is often described as a predominantly rural country (Donahue 1986). However, there has been increasing urbanization due to internal migration of the population from the rural areas to the cities. The political instability of the 1970s and 80s has accelerated this trend, and the proportion of the population living in a setting broadly defined as urban in 1985 was between 55 and 60 per cent (MINVAH, 1987*a*). This demographic shift is particularly noticeable in Managua, the capital city, where burgeoning settlements of self-made housing are one of the arresting features of the urban landscape.

In 1979, Nicaragua's health sector was typical of countries of comparable economic development. It included a hospital sector, administering hospitals in the capital and the provincial towns which accepted public and paying patients. A social security system was established in 1957 to provide care to government workers and to the insured work-force from Nicaragua's small manufacturing sector. This covered less than 10 per cent of the total population. The Ministry of Health was responsible for basic preventive programmes, such as childhood immunization and MCH, and also provided curative care to rural areas and the uninsured town dwellers. About twenty other locally-based agencies existed to address broadly defined health and social welfare problems (Garfield and Williams 1989).

The Nicaraguan health system prior to 1979 had been characterized as fragmented and disorganized (Donahue 1986), leading to inefficient service delivery to the population. This particularly affected the poorer and more marginal sectors of the community. The service developed reactively to needs as they arose. In this Nicaragua was no different from most developing countries, since the discourse around proactive planning for health in developing countries was a product of the 1960s, and was still awaiting implementation during the late 1970s.

As with many developing countries the direction of health sector policy and planning was heavily influenced by multilateral and bilateral agencies. Until 1979, the dominant external interest was the United States, either through charitable foundations or the state sponsored US Agency for International Development (USAID). Early public health campaigns and initiatives were supported by bodies such as the Rockefeller Foundation in the 1920s and 30s. The Pan-American Sanitary Bureau, prior to its incorporation into the World Health Organization, had a long history of involvement in public health interventions in Nicaragua.

In the 1960s, when comprehensive health planning came to the fore on the international health agenda, the Nicaraguan Ministry of Public Health, in co-operation with the Pan-American Health Organization, prepared the first National Health Plan for the ten-year period up until 1975. This plan was based on the received international strategy of the time, which saw improvements to the health of developing country populations coming through health services development and professional training. It aimed to increase coverage of these services, but urban services expanded and became more specialized, at the expense of basic rural health care. Reluctance of the trained professionals to go to rural areas and work for more than a short time was a major factor in Latin American countries (de Kadt 1982).

CHWS BEFORE THE REVOLUTION

By 1976, when the Second National Health Plan was drawn up, international health policy had shifted its focus. Basic health care services for rural areas had become prioritized over increasing the technical sophistication of urban health services. Pressure to reorientate Nicaragua's health policy and planning towards this issue came at a seminar of senior Nicaraguan Ministry of Health Officials and USAID representatives, held in Chinandega, Nicaragua, in 1976. This led to the second National Health Plan to fund three health programmes, which were targeted on the rural areas. One programme funded a rural health organizer, whose tasks were to recruit, train and support volunteer rural health collaborators. This was the first recognition in the formal health system of CHWs who had not received professional training, and who were not salaried employees of a health agency (Donahue 1986). Programmes training volunteer CHWs were enthusiastically supported by the non-governmental organizations which had been working in health programmes in rural areas for some years.

There were a number of such programmes organized through the voluntary sector which had been running for some years. Typical was a Nicaraguan-funded voluntary organization (PROVADENIC), connected to the private, religious Bautista Hospital. This had been supporting similar programmes for a number of years, as part of community development projects in alliance with various non-governmental agencies, often in association with religious organizations (C. Farren, personal communication).

In parallel to the services provided by the formal health system, an informal sector had traditionally addressed health needs of the Nicaraguan population. The two prominent practitioners in this sector were *curanderos* (traditional healers) and *parteras* (traditional birth attendants). Both worked from healing systems whose concepts lay outside those of Western biomedicine, though many of their practices eclectically incorporated its rituals.

The 1976 rural health programmes sought to train *parteras* as a

CHWs (Heiby 1982). As well as hygienic obstetric practice, they were to be trained in the provision of antenatal care, family planning, and the treatment of common childhood illnesses. The large scale programme trained 768 *parteras* at 47 courses during 1976 to 1978. At the end of the programme 497 *parteras* were continuing to contact programme officers for the resupply of medicines. However, this programme did not continue after 1979, with political instability cited as a major reason. The success or otherwise of this initiative has been debated (Habicht 1982).

In contrast, *curanderos* were not integrated into more general CHW programmes, the Nicaraguan experience being similar to that found in other developing countries (American Public Health Association 1977).

THE POLITICAL MOVEMENT AND THE STRUGGLE FOR HEALTH

The decade of the 1970s was a turbulent epoch for Nicaragua. The repressive and corrupt Somoza regime, in power dynastically since 1934, was entering its final phase. The earthquake in 1972, which had destroyed the capital Managua, provoked a crisis in the Somoza regime from which it never recovered. Internal pressure for political reform was exacerbated by the economic pressures affecting developing countries without oil. In Nicaragua the quiescence of the formal opposition through the years of the Somoza dictatorship meant that the Frente Sandinista de Liberacion Nacional (FSLN), a small clandestine cadre party, could skilfully exploit the political conjuncture (Black 1982).

However, to mobilize mass support in the anti-Somoza struggle, a structure was needed to widen the popular base. Development of the mass organizations provided the mechanism to reach the population. Mass organizations have been categorized into class-based organizations (such as trade unions for manual and agricultural workers) and non-class-based organizations, the most prominent of which were the Neighbourhood Committees (CDS) and the women's organization, AMPRONAC (now AMNLAE). The political programme of the FSLN was committed to the use of mass organizations in the tasks of overthrowing the dictatorship and in the processes involved in the subsequent reconstruction (Ruchwarger 1985).

Health demands have been an important propaganda component of revolutionary movements' wider social programmes. The FSLN did not need to prefigure the post-revolutionary scenario by detailed statements on health plans, beyond support for general demands such as free medical assistance to the entire population. The two main health organizations involved in the anti-Somoza struggle were the health workers' trade union (FETSALUD) and the doctors medical association (FESOMENIC). A Popular Medical Commission was established in 1978 to co-ordinate organized health workers in this fight (Consejo Nacional Popular de Salud 1984). After the 1979 revolution these groupings became important voices on behalf of their members in determining the direction of post-revolutionary health policy.

Community health work in rural communities was not seen as political activity opposed to the state by the Somoza government. This resulted in CHW programmes being targeted by the Ministry of Health on areas in which the 'guerrilla' operated, as a tactic to weaken support for the revolutionary movement and win support for the Somoza regime through the provision of health services. Ironically, many of the CHWs opposed the regime and welcomed the safe cover afforded by their role to move unmolested through the community (Donahue 1986).

Following the revolution in 1979, the new government embarked upon comprehensive reconstruction. The economic framework was to be a mixed economy divided into two main sectors, the private sector, where much of the agricultural production for export remained, and the public sector. Within the public sector the government's declared priorities were: first, defence; second, production and its encouragement through a programme of agrarian reform; third, education and in particular the reduction of the high levels of illiteracy; and fourth, health services.

The motor to achieve these was to be a strong central state, which would plan the development of comprehensive services throughout the country through professionally run, but politically controlled, ministries. A Ministry of Planning was established to co-ordinate strategy at a central level, and a normative planning methodology was applied to all ministries (Wilson 1987).

A more devolved approach based on local government was

initially precluded, as the Somoza regime had left no viable tier of regional administration. The development of a regional administrative structure to permit decentralization was one of the major political objectives of the early 1980s.

Central to the development plan was a framework of participative democracy in which the mass organizations were to play the key role. This, it was hoped, would counterbalance the vertical nature of the centralized development plan driven by ministerial functionaries and professionals.

The Health Ministry (MINSA) was reorganized and the many agencies contributing to national and local health services programmes came under its control. The government was committed to a national health service, the Sistema Nacional Unico de Salud (MINSA 1980). Its principles accorded with the spirit of the Alma Ata declaration and the policy of the Government of Reconstruction, in that the community was to be involved at all levels. This was explicitly stated in the policy statement.

The responsibilities of the Health Ministry included curative and preventive services and environmental health. The prime responsibilities for key determinants of public health, such as water and nutrition, lay with their respective ministries, the Ministry of Agriculture and Agrarian Reform (MIDINDRA), and the Ministry of Water Supply and Drainage (INAA). These were structured in the same way as the Health Ministry, with strong central control. Such a national structure for planning and implementation meant that intersectoral collaboration between agencies at the local level was vital if comprehensive PHC in its widest sense was to be achieved.

The first few years after 1979 saw the implementation of the remaining parts of the 1976 Health Plan. Broadly, this consisted of developing the secondary health care infrastructure in the regions by building four hospitals and expanding the primary care network through a programme of building health centres and health posts. From 1979 to 1985 the number of health centres more than doubled, increasing from 172 to 487 (Donahue 1986). A wide-ranging manpower training programme was implemented to train all categories of health professionals, in particular, auxiliary nurses and doctors, with the intake of medical students rising from 50 per annum to over 400 (Braverman and Roemer 1985). There were no initial plans to train CHWs.

To implement these plans an efficient management system was needed to ensure delivery of the newly developed service. A normative, target-setting, planning mechanism was used, which drew heavily from the planning and managment model of Cuba. Norms of practice were declared for each aspect of a programme and precise targets specified for each measurable component of activity. A review structure between regional and central levels was introduced in 1982 (MINSA 1983). While the regional tier maintained responsibilities for hospital services, the community services were developed by health areas. The final devolution of administrative responsibilities was to health areas, into which each regional health authority was divided.

In 1983, the comprehensive PHC programme, Programa Integral de Atencion en las Areas de Salud' (PIAAS) was implemented throughout the country (MINSA 1982*a*). This integrated and standardized the health services at the primary care level. The health services team covered curative services, enviromental health, local health education, community nursing services, and preventive programmes, such as immunization, growth-monitoring, and family planning. Each health area had a management team, led by the director, who was usually, though not exclusively, the doctor. In distant rural areas, this post was occasionally filled by a recent medical graduate performing statutory social service prior to receiving national registration to practice.

VOLUNTEERS FOR COMMUNITY HEALTH

In the post-1979 period in Nicaragua, community participation through volunteering to support health programmes was a major feature. The forms of volunteering were either as a one-day volunteer in one-day mass campaigns (*jornada brigadistas*), or in the more extended role of the PHC *brigadista*, which was the term for the CHWs (Scholl 1985). These roles and their evolution will be described.

Volunteers in one-day health campaigns (*jornada brigadistas*)

Immediately following the triumph of the revolution, the Health Ministry was concerned that outbreaks of infectious diseases could follow the civil war, during which there had been a breakdown of routine preventive services. In response, a number of one-day campaigns to vaccinate children took place, which recruited volunteers from the mass organizations who worked in conjunction with Health Ministry staff. The initial small campaigns developed to be country-wide mass campaigns in 1981 and 1982.

The Health Ministry defined the public health objectives for the campaigns (for example, vaccination, malaria eradication, environmental hygiene) and directed the technical operation (for example, ensuring the cold chain was maintained). To co-ordinate the campaigns within the Health Ministry, the Division of Education and Popular Communication (DECOPS) was established as a division in its own right. Out of mass organizations came the Popular Health Commissions (later Councils) which participated in the planning and co-ordination. These Councils were established at national, regional, and area level, and liaised with ministry staff in DECOPS. Health education and training materials were prepared nationally as a joint venture between the popular educators in the Ministry and the representatives of the mass organizations. For each campaign, cartoon pamphlets were used for training volunteers and were printed and distributed in two out of the three national newspapers.

These pamphlets were developed by DECOPS following popular workshops, and explained the scientific and technical background to any given campaign in a manner which attempted to demystify its complexities (Donahue 1986). The mass organizations were vital in the recruitment of volunteers for the campaign and in co-ordinating training. Local workshops were held for training and a multiplier system was used, whereby the initial training sessions prepared trainers to cascade skills. The subjects of the one-day campaigns were childhood vaccination (mainly non-injectable polio vaccine), mass drug administration for malaria, environmental hygiene and first aid (Coordination Nacional de las Jornadas Populares de Salud 1984). The style of the campaigns and their predominantly disease specific targets followed in the tradition of many previous initiatives in the Pan-American Health Organization region in the last forty years (Williams 1988). However, the level of participation was unprecedented.

The one-day health campaigns were widely supported. For example, in 1981 over 28 000 *brigadistas* were trained from 1815 workshops, using 5592 trainers for the polio campaign. Similar rates of involvement were found for the campaign to improve environmental hygiene (Coordination Nacional de las Jornadas Populares de Salud 1984). The campaign which involved the greatest number of participants was the mass drug administration against malaria. This campaign trained 77 000 *brigadistas*, which was approximately one *brigadista* for every thirty in the population (Garfield and Vermund 1983).

The socio-demographic characteristics were surveyed from 30 000 volunteers who participated in a one-day environmental hygiene campaign in 1982. Two-thirds of the *brigadistas* were women, mostly housewives or students; of the male *brigadistas* the majority were either rural farmers or urban students. Only 20 per cent of brigadistas were salaried workers or self-employed. 75 per cent were under 25 years of age, and 20 per cent under 15 years (MINSA 1982*b*).

Most major campaigns took place during the weekend, which allowed maximum opportunity for employed workers to participate. The factors which ensure administrative success were efficient central organization, good liaison between the Health Ministry and community organizations, and mass popular support. In a country with remote pockets of population, the provision of State-owned vehicles to transport the *brigadistas* on the days of the campaigns demonstrated the value of intersectoral collaboration.

Support for the campaigns was not uniform throughout Nicaragua. Coverage by the campaigns in any given area was dependent upon the support of the local population for the mass organizations. In Special Zone II, on the Atlantic Coast, the mass organizations had a weak base. This meant that only 1 in 125 persons trained as *brigadistas* in the mass drug administration campaign against malaria. However, in this area, the annual rate of malaria cases presenting to health services was ten times that of the Pacific Coast area of Esteli, where participation was highest. This was a major difficulty in making one day campaigns based on popular participation effective (Garfield and Vermund 1986).

Participation in the campaigns in the early years became a symbol of the continued success of the revolution, with personal participation being considered evidence of support for the revolutionary process. Invitations to participate in the campaigns by the national media mixed political imperative with moral overtones, a style reported in relation to the mass health education campaigns carried out in Cuba in the 1970s (Tesh 1986).

Since the campaigns were not carried out as controlled interventions, it is impossible to evaluate formally their effectiveness. In the malaria campaign the objective of eradication was not achieved, though a reduction in the number of cases reported to health services was observed. In the months following the campaign, however, no long-term reduction was observed (Garfield and Vermund 1983). Similar results have been seen following attempts to apply mass drug administration elsewhere (Bruce-Chwatt 1983).

There is no doubt that the one-day campaigns gave a significant boost to the continuing programmes of the Health Ministry in raising vaccine uptake and minimizing malaria. The campaigns contributed to increasing uptake of polio vaccination levels, and in the period 1983–88 there were no reported cases of acute poliomyelitis. In the five years prior to 1979, there were between 20 and 40 cases notified annually to MINSA.

Potential disadvantages of the one day campaigns have been their short-term nature, the disruption of routine for full-time health workers and the alienation of the medical profession, leading to their obstructing programme implementation (Garfield and Williams 1989).

CHWs: the extended role for the PHC *brigadista*

The CHW programmes introduced into the 1976 Health Plan were omitted when it was revitalized by the Health Ministry after the 1979 revolution. However, the success of a national campaign to improve literacy served as a fillip to extend the role of volunteering in health beyond the one-day campaigns.

In 1980, the Ministry of Education, with sponsorship of UNESCO, carried out a literacy campaign using mainly school and college students. These educators went for five months to rural communities, where they taught reading and writing skills to those disadvantaged by poor or non-existent services during the previous regime (Miller 1985). The success of this campaign, both in its objectives and in its involvement of the mass organizations, made the repetition of its success in the field of health a political objective, which outranked the Ministry's priority to develop services based on salaried professionals.

By the end of 1981 the Health Ministry had drawn up a comprehensive PHC plan in conjunction with the Pan-American Health Organization, which included a key role for a volunteer CHW, who would work alongside the professional workers in health areas (MINSA 1982*a*). They were called PHC *brigadistas*. Most of those recruited for training had participated in one-day campaigns. The only requirement for selection of a CHW was literacy or current enrolment in an adult literacy class.

Within the Health Ministry the Division of Education and Popular Communication (DECOPS), the department which had co-ordinated the one-day campaigns, was responsible for the implementation of programmes of training for the extended role of the CHW. They were to be managed by the Popular Educator who was a salaried employee of the Ministry and a member of the Primary Health Care Team. The role of the Popular Educator was to recruit, organize, train, and motivate the CHWs with the support of the Popular Health Council. Many of the Popular Educators had been particularly committed one-day campaigners. Regional Popular Educators had frequently worked with DECOPS in the ministry.

With the PHC plan (PIAAS) the main tasks outlined for the CHW were extensive in scope: health education in the community, co-operation with the preventive programmes, treatment of simple illness, and faciliation of patient referral to professionally staffed health posts and administrative functions. By September 1983, 33 out of 97 health areas had trained such CHWs (Scholl 1985).

The role of these CHWs (PHC *brigadistas*) has been discussed in case studies from two sites on the Pacific Coast and the remote Atlantic Coast in Special Zone II. The role of the CHW in two rural health areas on the Pacific Coast was found to be limited (Scholl 1985). Though managerially the CHWs were responsible to the Popular Educator, most of the curative and educational tasks were carried out by the CHW under the guidance of the auxiliary nurse. In one setting the CHW supported the auxiliary nurse in clinic activities and participated in the rota for staffing health centre departments, such as equipment preparation units, injection, and wound dressing. In these activities, the role was close to one of being 'just another pair of hands' (Walt 1990).

Information collecting was one of the tasks that fell to the CHW following the introduction of PHC programmes. Vertically integrated plans demanded that data were collected and collated as part of the preparation of local health profiles. A key part of the PIAAS plan was, that for each sector in a health area a small booklet of local information was prepared concerning demography, housing, main employers, and prominent environmental health hazards, which would contribute to preparing a community diagnosis. In many areas the community health volunteers were assigned the task of collecting the information. As many were school students, this work fitted in with the school curriculum, which demanded that projects relevant to their local community should be undertaken. Some authors have argued that this role allowed research methods to be demystified (Fals-Borda 1987). This may have been the case, but many CHWs saw this as delegation of irksome, low status administration, while the auxiliary nurses concentrated on clinical care. CHWs who carried out a wider role also existed. However, this was a rare exception, attributed to the charismatic individual who had profound links with the community and the local political system.

On the Atlantic Coast of Nicaragua, where rural villages were often remote from the local health centre, there was a clear need to train and equip CHWs for the wider role envisaged by the PIAAS plan (Donahue 1986; Ellesberg 1982).

In this region, known as Special Zone II until 1988, and now as the Region Autonoma Atlantico Sur, the extended role of CHWs must be understood in its political context. The Atlantic Coast had not participated in the overthrow of the Somoza Regime, and consequently there was limited support for the government of reconstruction. The local population was not receptive to the development of mass organizations around overt political issues. This was reflected in the low participation rates in the one-day (*jornada*) campaigns discussed above. However, health was seen as an important conduit for integrating the population into the revolutionary process. For this reason, along with the remoteness, the Regional Health Ministry prioritized Popular Education Programmes in the rural areas. CHWs were not recruited instead of professional workers. Even in the remotest part of Special Zone II a fully staffed professional health post was never more than 30 miles away, with a full complement of doctor, graduate nurse, and supporting auxiliaries usually doing their compulsory social service.

In remote health areas, such as La Cruz del Rio Grande and

Tortugero, where the population was widely dispersed, there was scope for the wider role. However, in the health areas where there were small town settlements, such as Kukra Hill and Lagunda de Perlas, the role of the CHW was similar to that on the Pacific Coast, and was fulfilled, in the main, by secondary school students (Coyle 1983). The Regional Health Ministry sanctioned the distribution of medicines and supplies to trained CHWs who lived in remote communities. This went against the general policy of MINSA and contrasted with the restricted access, for fear of leakage to Contra forces, of medicines to nurses in the main health centre in the regional capital, Bluefields. During periodic refresher courses for CHWs and *parteras* in Bluefields, medicines were obtained from two sources, through restocking their emergency supplies, and by obtaining medicines ostensibly for personal and family use following consultation with the Ministry's doctors at the Bluefields Health Centre.

In Special Zone II, the majority of the CHWs recruited were not from the English-speaking members of the black population nor the indigenous ethnic groups (Miskito and Rama). Combined these groups constituted over 60 per cent of the population of this region (MINVAH 1987*b*). 80 per cent of CHWs were recruited from Spanish speakers, most of whom had emigrated to the region in the previous twenty years (Comision Popular de La Salud, Zona Especial II 1984).

The effectiveness of this strategy was not lost on anti-government forces operating on the Atlantic Coast, who saw all health personnel, including CHWs as important targets in their destructive campaign to erode the social base of the Government after the revolution (Garfield 1989). The immunity that health workers had enjoyed in the early 1970s in developing countries, from their perceived apolitical role, had vanished by the 1980s, as health became a high-profile plank of the government's social programme (Heggenhougen 1984).

Training and motivation

Where CHW programmes existed, training courses for CHW *brigadistas* prepared them for a wide repertoire of roles, curative, preventive, and promotional. These courses used their own materials prepared by DECOPS and the work of David Werner (Werner and Bower 1982). Organization of courses was the responsibility of the regional and area Popular Educators. The primary courses took up to five days with periodic refresher courses lasting one day. The classes were small (less than twenty), used an interactive workshop format in preference to didactic lectures, and made full use of expressive educational techniques, called socio-drama. These courses contrasted in length and in content with those provided by the Ministry for auxiliary nurses. These lasted nine months and the curriculum was dominated by the Ministry's programme norms. Classes were large (up to one hundred) and the teaching style was, by necessity, didactic.

One interesting aspect of volunteering is the motivation of those who do it, and the context within which participation occurs. In the early period following the revolution, the desire to contribute to the reconstruction attracted many to support the health campaigns. To those who stand outside a revolutionary period of history such altruism may seem hard to credit. The strength and sustainability of revolutionary voluntarism has been described in other developing countries following a national and social revolution (White 1983). The health campaigns found broad support even from those who did not ascribe to the political objectives of the FSLN. To be a one-day *brigadista* for health was to participate in the revolution. Indeed, the Health Ministry's slogan printed on all its stationery was 'revolution is health'.

However, few incentives beyond revolutionary commitment existed for those who took on the demanding role of the extended *brigadista*. Occasionally, preferential access to the limited medicines, for the CHW and the family, available at a health facility occurred. CHW work was sanctioned by the school curricula as suitable activity for Work and Study courses, which form part of the core curriculum of post-primary education. This specific incentive may explain why adolescents made up the largest proportion of one-day volunteers. Successful completion of these programmes was taken into consideration when applying for professional training in the health sector.

Even in the professional health service there were few material incentives for improved performance. At all levels of Nicaraguan society the emulation system was introduced. This was a system where high-performing workers were distinguished in front of their colleagues at a formal work-related ceremony, where material rewards were occasionally given. A similar system of incentives has been described in the productive sector of the bureaucratic collectivist states, which existed in Eastern Europe (Nove 1983).

Parteras empiricas: traditional birth attendants

The limited role given to CHWs by the implementation of the PIAAS programme could not be enforced on the traditional birth attendants (*parteras empiricas*). Their attendance at over 60 per cent of all births in Nicaragua cut deep into the territory that the Health Ministry wished its services and newly trained professionals to occupy. The official MINSA policy was that all births should be attended in a Ministry institution by a doctor, though lack of resources and women's preferences continues to make that goal unlikely to be achieved in the short to medium term.

Therefore, the programme for the training of the *parteras* developed in the 1976 National Plan (Heiby 1982) was not initially revived. In 1981, the Esteli Health Region supported a programme of contacting, organizing, and training *parteras*. The success of this project, which fitted in with the UNICEF International Programme, led the Ministry to accept that in the medium term the integration of the *parteras* was a necessary policy and regions were encouraged to implement training programmes in 1984 (Veraguas 1984).

Planned expansion of CHW programmes

By late 1984, with PIAAS now fully implemented, DECOPS recognized that the role of the community health volunteer had not developed as had been hoped (Scholl 1985). An attempt was made to put forward a new scheme which trained the CHWs for specialized roles. These were sanitary worker, primary care worker, mother and child health worker, school health *brigadista*, occupational health *brigadista* and *partera*. Implementation was limited, despite DECOPS attempts to reach agreement within the Ministry to redefine the working relationship of the CHW. Although new roles were accepted on paper, the relationship on the ground was dictated by control of roles which remained firmly in the hands of the salaried professional workers, in particular the auxiliary nurses.

THE FURTHER DEVELOPMENT OF CHW PROGRAMMES

Intended development of CHW programmes was hindered by the intensification of the US-backed attacks by the Contra forces upon Nicaragua. Up to the end of 1987, nearly a quarter of the 600 health facilities in Nicaragua had been destroyed, damaged or closed down by Contra activity (Garfield 1989). The *brigadistas* were considered legitimate targets by the opposition forces, with more than 40 being killed and more being kidnapped or threatened. Some have been forced to work with the Contras or, at least, supply them with medicines and equipment (Garfield and Williams 1989).

This intimidation had severe effects upon the running of CHW programmes. In Special Zone II, for example, the number of functioning *brigadistas* fell from 250 in 1983 to 60 in 1984 following such attacks. When the military threat decreased the numbers recovered, up to 120 in 1986 (Garfield and Williams 1989). Vaccination campaigns were sometimes held unannounced, prior to the officially designated day, so as to avoid Contra activity. Household visits would have to be arranged, so people could not be attacked on the way to clinics.

However, the decrease in activity has not only been caused by Contra attacks. The general level of population participation in the Nicáraguan political system has declined since the early days of the revolution. The Sandinista Defence Committees (CDS), the main locus of community based participation, had over 700 000 members in the early 1980s, but this had declined to 150 000 by 1987 (Close 1988).

The reasons for this shrinkage were not just an example of the demoralizing effects of the war. Commandante Leticia Herrera, the FSLN member in charge of the CDS, noted that they had a tendency to become authoritarian arms of the State, with purely executive function (Ruchwarger 1985). This decline in the level of participatory democracy, together with the tendency for the mass organizations to become merely the channel for centralized decision making of the government and ruling party, have been seen as key elements in the fall in popularity of the FSLN, which culminated in the electoral defeat in February 1990 (Tucker 1989; Gonzalez 1990).

Participation in the Popular Health Councils and the *brigadista* programmes have generally continued to decline despite the reduction in the intensity of Contra attacks. In one health district in Managua, the number of volunteers decreased from around 1200 in 1987 to less than 800 in 1989. The activities of these volunteers were largely confined to performing the censuses required before vaccination campaigns, a task taking up several weekends of work, and then, on vaccination days, supporting the establishment of vaccination posts and transporting clients to them. In early 1990, there was an energetic campaign to recruit more volunteers for vaccination programmes which constituted a key element in MINSA's prioritized activity 'the campaign for the defence of the life of the child'. Following the electoral defeat of the FSLN, however, many volunteers withdrew from what was still seen as partly political work.

CONCLUSION

The Nicaraguan experience with CHWs has been considered to be special, and to have transcended some of the inherent limitations of the PHC strategy. Political direction is the crucial element in this respect. It has been stated that 'political commitment, sometimes under adverse conditions may . . . unite and stimulate voluntary effort, as witnessed Nicaragua' (Walt 1990). In this chapter we have discussed both the successs and the limitations of the Nicaraguan CHW programmes, and have attempted to evaluate whether the Nicaraguan experience is one which should be considered a model for CHW programmes elsewhere.

The initial policy of the Health Ministry (MINSA) after the revolution was to develop a doctor-centred, curative health service, run in conjunction with public health programmes. It is arguable that this policy was ostensibly less progressive with regard to CHWs than the policy on paper of the outgoing government. The declared preference for the high-profile health services development reflected the policy commitment of the FSLN during its struggle for power. Commitment to accessible health care by the FSLN was an important propaganda feature during this period. Concentration upon low technology, appropriate health care by the post-revolutionary government could have been interpreted as offering second-rate health care. Lay knowledge within Nicaragua views the biomedical model of US health services as the pinnacle of excellence.

The PHC programme (PIAAS) launched by the Health Ministry in 1983 included a key role for a CHW to work alongside the professional members of the health team. The potential for the development of a CHW with a wide scope indicated in the programme was not realized on its implementation in 1983. While the intention of the PHC programme was to provide a coherent framework to strengthen PHC, its implementation in 1983 was rapid and vertical. Team integration and community engagement were sacrificed for standardized delivery of vertically defined programmes. Such a rigid approach gave neither flexibility for professional staff, nor the environment to develop the CHW. Far from being autonomous, the CHW was at the end of a long line of command.

The use of CHW *brigadistas* in Nicaragua in the period 1982–83, when the PIAAS plan was being implemented, varied from region to region. Volunteer CHW programmes were developed depending on regional ministry enthusiasm and mass organization interest locally. Some regions had little enthusiasm, despite a predominantly rural population. In other regions, the regional Health Ministry saw CHW programmes as a marginal issue, and thus there was little interference, resulting in considerable flexibility for Popular Health Educators. The experience in Special Zone II showed that there could be flexibility in the centrally driven normative PHC plan being implemented in 1983. In Special Zone II, remoteness and the particular political situation meant that CHWs were permitted to carry out the wider role for which they had been trained. Interestingly, the high level of activity of PHC *brigadistas* was accompanied by a low level of participation in the one-day campaigns. That the extended role of the CHW as envisaged in PIAAS was still limited was demonstrated in this region, where implementation was most complete.

At a more general level, an inhibiting factor to the CHW programme development may have been the experiences of leading members of the FSLN during the guerrilla wars, when medical and surgical care by doctors was vital in the treatment of casualties. In addition, the FSLN had obligations to professional health workers, whose organizations had been participants in the anti-Somoza struggle. Both FETSALUD and the Medical Association had precise demands for the post-revolutionary health plan to focus upon developing health services to be staffed by a professional, salaried work-force. These aspirations coincided with the economic policy of the reconstructon period to integrate the adult population into formal employment. Volunteer programmes which extended beyond one-day commitment ran directly counter to this.

An indirect source of inhibition came from the strong presence at all levels of the health system of Cuban advisors. The Cuban health model, focusing upon technological medicine delivered through a doctor-led vertical management system, found the unpaid CHW programme alien to its experience.

The early strategy, with only a small role for CHWs, was modified as the revolutionary process developed. This was partly in response to pressure from volunteers involved in the one day campaigns and the cadre of community organizers which had developed around DECOPS in the Health Ministry. This coincided with the intentions of the FSLN to use the mass organization in participatory democracy. With notable exceptions, however, the expanded role for the CHW remained largely unfulfilled. This was partly due to the political and military attacks upon Nicaragua while the FSLN was in power. The political opposition within Nicaragua attempted to sabotage the mass campaigns by releasing propaganda against vaccines and medicines used. Propaganda against these campaigns was broadcast from Contra radio stations. Military attacks and threats were also directed at CHWs and at campaign organizers. Community participation in health programmes was thought to lead to increased support and involvement with the government of reconstruction, and therefore became a key target for Contra attacks.

The attacks upon the health system were successful at several levels. There were large outbreaks of controllable infectious diseases, such as malaria and measles, especially in war affected areas (Garfield and Williams 1989; Garfield *et al.* 1989). The war also meant that hospital casualty services became a prioritized area for health care. This led to a focus on curative hospital services, with corresponding limitation of resources to the PHC programme. The level of participation in health collapsed after the intensification of the opposition struggle against the Sandinista government. While this was partly due to direct attacks upon volunteers, the greater success of the Contra strategy was to destablize the Nicaraguan economy. This led to a fall in the support enjoyed by the FSLN, and participation in the political and revolutionary process fell generally, including the health sector.

With the election of the new government in the spring of 1990, Nicaraguan history continues to change rapidly. It is too early to report on the effects of this change upon health policy and the level of community participation, although the prospects are clearly not bright (Hopkinson and Chalmers 1990). The implications of the Nicaraguan experience with CHWs concern more general debates, however. This chapter has identified that even when the political will was present at the highest government level, the implementation of PHC programmes still resulted in only a limited role for CHWs. It is not adequate, therefore, to cite lack of political support as a sufficient explanation, when accounting for the generally disappointing outcomes of CHW programmes.

9

The village context of Honduras' VHW programme: 1980–84

CARL KENDALL

INTRODUCTION

In the early 1970s, Honduras, one of the poorest countries in the Western hemisphere, established a rural-focused innovative, primary health care (PHC) system. The Ministry of Health (MOH) has pursued a policy of encouraging village-level participation in its programme. As a document prepared for Health Sector Planning (Agency for International Development 1977) pointed out:

> In 1973, the Ministry of Health initiated implementation of a policy of extension of coverage of health and sanitation programs into the rural areas. The program is based on a regionalized system of levels of care ranging from community volunteers, through auxiliary nurse dispensaries, to national hospitals. The overall policy of extension of coverage corresponds to the model of using integrated rural health services to reach the poor majority.

Health problems in Honduras

The country faced enormous health needs. The Plan Nacional de Dessarrollo: Plan Nacional de Salud 1979–1983 (National Development Plan: National Health Plan 1979–1983, referred to here as the PNS) noted the lamentable health conditions found in Honduras, especially in rural areas. Citing the Encuesta Demografico Nacional de Honduras (EDENH) of 1972 (Honduran National Demographic Census), the PNS noted that Honduras had (and still has) the third highest crude mortality rate (14.2/1000), and the third highest infant mortality rate (117.0/1000 live births) in Latin America and the

Caribbean. These figures rise if only rural Honduras is considered (16.5/1000 and 127.2/1000 live births respectively).

These rates were the highest in Central America, and are, for the most part, due to infectious diseases. For example, diarrhoea and accompanying dehydration was the single largest known cause of death (12.4 per cent in 1972, 12.2 per cent in 1974 (Direccion General de Estadistica y Censos 1980), and the single largest cause of infant death. In 1977, diarrhoeal disease was attributed as the cause in 1030 infant deaths. This constituted 24.4 per cent of the 4227 recorded infant deaths. The 110 393 cases of diarrhoea recorded in the MOH, Honduras Division of Biostatistics in 1978 signifies a crude morbidity rate of 3210.6/100 000 persons. Were this to be age-adjusted, the actual occurrence of diarrhoea in small children would be perceived to be pandemic. Because of oral rehydration solution and home-based strategies for prevention, diagnosis and treatment, acute dehyrating diarrhoeas appear to be amenable to PHC outreach activities, and the active involvement of VHWs.

Institutional health care and community participation

The MOH has developed a system of institutional and geographic levels for referral of health problems from the community to the national hospital. Five levels of cosmopolitan, or institutional, health care exist. At the apex stand the six national hospitals, responsible for physician training, the performance of especially difficult procedures, and care of the chronically and mentally ill. At the next lowest level are the regional hospitals, medium-sized hospitals where most patients are treated; next are area hospitals, previously emergency hospitals of about 50 beds. Below this level are the municipal health services. These are the CESAMO, or Centro de Salud Medico (Physician-staffed Health Centre), and the CESAR, or Centro de Salud Auxiliar (Auxiliary Nurse-staffed Centre.

Only the municipal level co-ordinates community participation in health programmes. Based at the CESAMOs and CESARs are rural Health Promoters, responsible, for the most part, for water and sanitation projects. The CESAR is staffed by an Auxiliary Nurse, who receives eleven months of instruction. In each rural village (*aldea*) a Health Guardian (HG) provides simple home-based care and a Health Representative (HR) co-ordinates community con-

Table 9.1 Ministry of Health facilities, 1981

National hospitals	5
Regional hospitals	6
CESAMOs	95
CESARs	433

struction activities. The HG is envisioned as the village level counterpart of the Auxiliary Nurse, and MOH personnel have emphasized the selection of women. The HR is the counterpart of the Health Promoter, and men are preferred. Neither the HG nor the HR are paid employees of the MOH, and are supposed to be volunteers elected by their communities for participation. In addition, midwives have been trained by the MOH to provide birthing services in many communities.

However, the difficulties the MOH has faced in Honduras are well known. In 1981, the MOH had 465 centres, including 19 hospitals, and a salaried staff of 8199 (see Table 9.2). The number of hospitals exceeds the optimistic goals set for 1983 by the PNS for national and regional hospitals, and has fulfilled goals for CESAMOs and CESARs.

The difficulties relate to the imbalance between village-level staff and permanent staff, as well as to the costs of the fixed facilities and permanent staff, which have been compounded in this decade. As

Table 9.2 Ministry of Health personnel, 1981

Salaried staff		*Active volunteer staff*	
(Unidad de Investigacion y Desarrollo Administrativo) June 1981			
Physicians	812	Midwives	503
Nurses	338	Guardians	296
Auxiliary Nurses	2708	Representatives	251
Technicians	900	Total	1050
Health Inspectors	336		
Health Promoters	196		
Administrative	2909		
Total	8199		

Table 9.3 Ministry of Health estimated costs for fixed facilities and outreach programmes, 1983

Type of facility	No. of facilities anticipated	Cost of running the facility in Lempiras	Cost/ attention
National hospital	3	6 466 000	10.95
Regional hospital	6	15 537 000	8.76
Area hospital	21	7 476 000	6.57
CESAMO	92	9 085 800	4.38
CESAR	453	7 305 100	2.19
Institutional subtotal		45 871 300	5.14
Health Guardians	3600	901 700	0.42
Midwives	6000	135 000	0.38
Village level Health Workers		1 036 700	0.41
Total		46 908 000	4.10

Table 9.3 demonstrates, fully 99.8 per cent of the total Ministry health budget was to be spent on fixed facility programmes. This was projected, for the fiscal year 1983, to be a total of 45 871 300 Lempiras [2 Lempiras = $1 (1982)]. This figure is only the cost of running these facilities, not the capital cost associated with construction, overhead, and debt service. Increased hospital construction during the 1980s has only added to this cost burden.

Furthermore 29 480 400 Lempiras, or 62.8 per cent, of the total projected 1983 budget, were spent in expensive hospital care. As Table 9.3 shows, hospital care costs five times per patient what CESAR care costs (not including capital expenditure), and costs 27 times what VHW care costs.

Although the kinds of services offered by the national hospitals, and the cost of this care must of necessity differ, it must not be imagined that the hospitals treat only refractory cases or complicated illness. Since diarrhoea accounts for such a large proportion of all recorded diseases, all levels of health facility must treat it. Fully one-half of admissions of children under five to the teaching hospital in Tegucigalpa during 1978 were for dehydration that accompanied diarrhoea. Yet the treatment used in hospital is often the same oral rehydration solution found in the countryside.

Village health care

If hospital-based care is not the solution to these problems, do VHW programmes offer an alternative? The literature promoting PHC and the utilization of local-level health personnel is, for the most part, programmatic. Visionary applications of community development techniques and a facile co-option of local-level personnel are proposed. Most of the literature falls short, however, of dealing with the conflict inherent in such programmes. The decentralized nature of village-level health programmes and the emphasis on prevention found in community-based health programmes, often create intellectual and administrative problems for health authorities, and conflict between health ministries and villages.

Methods for planning the implementation of VHW programmes have also been inadequate. Uniform planning models and task assignments are often proposed from the capital, or through global programmes, and little in the way of active community involvement has been used. In the seminal aspect of workscope development and VHW recruitment, major global programmes have paid little attention.

An anthropologist, Gretchen Eoff (1980), conducted a study of three health regions in Honduras and made recommendations to the Ministry and Agency for International Development (AID). The Project Paper and programme planning for the VHW programme cited above (AID 1977) drew heavily on her conclusions. The report discussed geographical, economic, cognitive, and social factors in the utilization of MOH resources, and voiced some commonly held complaints against Ministry services. She argued that rural populations are, for the most part, willing to participate in MOH village-based programmes, but that failures of programme administration, logistical support, and Ministry resistance to rural country people's beliefs and conditions of life detract from Ministry success. Her report also discussed the cultural, economic and social gulf separating rural recipients of care and cosmopolitan healers, and the importance of integrating these beliefs and healers into the Ministry's programme. Eoff's argument had a common thread: the further the programme from cosmopolitan centres, and the lower the status of the health personnel and recipients, the less effective is the programme.

Many physicians found the discussion of the integration of native healers and village representatives into PHC too glib, however (Kendall 1984). These physicians are competing with local-level health personnel; they often feel the lives of their patients are jeopardized by local healers, and they resent the colonial implications of providing 'witch's' medicine. Few cosmopolitan health personnel seem willing to understand that the resistance to treatment modes, health education programmes, and co-operation with Ministry personnel is based on deeply felt alternative beliefs, tied to the organization and culture of the local rural environment (Wellin 1955; Paul 1958; Rubel 1964). Yet understanding health care seeking in the local environment, and rural country people's perceptions of urban-based programmes, is necessary for the MOH and health care personnel in general. It can be assumed that unless the MOH eschews extension of coverage, no other alternative health delivery scheme can be envisioned in the immediate future for Honduras.

Study design

The research presented here was part of a larger programme documented by Foote *et al.* (1985), and this chapter focuses on the socio-cultural context of VHW programme implementaton in Honduras. First, the rationale for the programme has been reviewed, and this is followed by discussion of the social and cultural features of thé Honduran countryside.

Finally, the case-study method of controlled comparison (Eggan 1954) is adapted to investigate the acceptance and utilization of VHWs in two sites where the programme has been implemented—the rural *aldeas* of Aqua Fresca and Los Dolores, situated some five miles apart.

Both *aldeas* share practically identical topographical features, rainfall, quantity and quality of naturally availale water sources, crops and cropping patterns, land tenure systems, and other economic, social, and cultural characteristics. Informants describe the physical characteristics of Aqua Fresca and Los Dolores as being much alike.

Both are visited by the same health workers and have access to the same CESAMO clinic of the MOH, but the two communities differ in terms of VHW acceptance and utilization. Aqua Fresca has an excellent village HG and HR, both part of the MOH extension programme since 1969. The village has a large number of houses with piped potable water, and has a number of latrines in use. The community participates actively in vaccination drives, attends health committee meetings, seems self-motivated with regard to health issues, and organizes easily for the purposes of health promotion. Los Dolores, on the other hand, has no HG, has an HR who participates only occasionally in Ministry activities, has constructed only two wells which operate only seasonally, and has no operating activities.

DESCRIPTION OF AQUA FRESCA AND LOS DOLORES

Aqua Fesca and Los Dolores are both villages in the municipality of Nance, a mountainous area in one of the 18 departments of Honduras, El Paraiso. The department is part of Health region I in the interior Highlands of Honduras which surrounds Tegucigalpa, and spreads south and east to encompass some 220 000 people.

The town centre is connected to Tegucigalpa by an all weather dirt road, and lies approximately 1½ hours from the capital. The town centre has a telegraph and telephone, as well as a CESAMO. The CESAMO is staffed by a physician, two nurses and a Health Promotor. One of the nurses is a local healer who has been successfully maintained in the Health Centre due to community pressure. There are three MOH trained midwives in Nance, as well as one midwife-masseuse who refused the training, and two *injectadores* who will inject medications brought to them by their clients.

Neither Aqua Fresca nor Los Dolores has a true centre, and houses are scattered close to fields throughout the extensive terrain of both villages. The geographic propinquity guarantees similarities of soil types, terrain, and rainfall, and the agricultural cycle varies little between the two communities in basic crops (corn, beans, sugar cane). Aqua Fresca, however, has an active resin co-operative which taps trees and provides cash income for a number of families. Los Dolores at one time supported resining and several families in Los Dolores still resin in nearby communities, but the activity was conducted on an individual basis, and failed to incorporate the community as a whole.

In both *aldeas* practically all household heads own property. Although patterns of ownership vary, the overwhelming pattern of *minifundia* is shared. In addition, almost all families possess animals—dogs, chickens, and pigs.

Local social organization

Mestizo or Ladino social organization has not been the subject of significant anthropological inquiry. An interpretive perspective applied to rural Ladino life is that of 'loose structure' (Kendall 1983). Rural country people seem to live in a 'rule-free' environment. Marriages seem transient, many 'illegitimate' children are born, inheritance is contested, individual disputes are resolved through violence, and voluntary organizations appear to form and dissolve rapidly.

The communities studied here, based on a core of consanguineous kin, can be considered, in an internal sense, closed and traditional, but do accept and sell land to outsiders. A traditional focus is found in the local emphasis on a strong leader, or *cacique*. Caciquismo, either on the local or the national level, is a persistent feature of Latin and Mediterranean society.

Country people are loosely organized into *parentelas*, or kin-based groups, but the local household, predominantly a conjugal family unit, is the elemental feature of social organization. Shared resources and claims on those resources among kin still spark many disputes and factions. On the other hand, country people travel frequently to town centres and the national capital to conduct business, and many parents have children who work in Tegucigalpa. Most households have radios, and each town has a battery-powered television. The possibilities of high geographical mobility, and the pressures induced by the high birth rate, guarantee that many parents and many children look for opportunities outside their village.

Differential distribution of wealth and power creates clashes and factions. Shared economic opportunities, shared local economy, shared household organization, and myriad details of social and economic organization bind local life. A shared history, patterns of resort, exposure to diverse traditions also guarantee similarities of response to programmes. What are these factors?

The household unit and kinship ties

The households of these villages are in both a normal and a normative sense conjugal family units. The husband, wife, and umarried offspring occupy a single house, and mean household size for the families studied in both villages is 5.83. This differs little from figures of the 1950s (Adams 1957) although it is somewhat different from those published in the Honduran census. The residence pattern may be established at marriage, if a formal marriage takes place, or at the birth of a child to the couple. Construction of a separate house, and provision of an independent hearth, constitutes the final solemnization of a marriage. Prior to this the husband and wife are a satellite household, usually within the husband's father's house.

Many people are mobile, however, and migrate for work, which has great implications for a VHW programme. In the community of Los Dolores, adult sons and daughters often decide to move. Of the 41 total households, 16 have children living outside, either temporarily or permanently, who regularly remit food, clothing, and money. This group constitutes 39 per cent of all households in Los Dolores.

Another group of 16 households have fostered grandchildren and other children, and 14 such households (87.5 per cent) receive regular remittances from the natural parents. Only four of these 16 households have fostered children who are not consanguineally related, and only two contain *hijos de crianza*, as these children are called; the other two have both *hijos de crianza* and fostered grandchildren. In the remaining two households non-resident children contribute regularly to household maintenance. The significance of family obligation in the absence of co-residence is clear. The fact that most parents who leave children in the households regularly contribute to their upkeep demonstrates the importance of these kin ties. Although children spend much time in households not of their immediate biological parents, in no way does this imply that their links with parents are severed, or that those parents do not maintain responsibility for their offspring.

Another point remains to be discussed. There is generally felt to be a great deal of desertion in marriage in Honduras. Of the 41 households in Los Dolores in 1981, there is no single example of a mature operating female-headed household. There are, of course, some elderly solitary females who live near family members, but these are clearly dependent households. This example demonstrates that, though the personnel may change, the form of the conjugal family unit, and sometimes the extended conjugal family, is maintained in Los Dolores. In most cases, the marriages have been quite stable, and although high rates of desertion and divorce can be expected in the first years of marriage, once in middle life the relationship stabilizes. The conjugal family unit, which we might anticipate from the categorical system of kinship, is, in fact, the form of household found in Honduras.

Hostility, disputes, and caquismo

The popular sociology of Ladino society is also replete with accounts of interpersonal hostility and competition, and the use of violence to settle disputes. In rural Honduras, this competition often takes place within the sibling group, and between partially related families. Primarily they can be regarded as events within a 'familiar' domain. Legal sanctions or procedures are rarely used to settle these disputes, which soon develop the character of feuds. The violence which may follow is often a terrible, tortured consequence of no-holds-barred, unsanctioned private actions. In short, it is an insider's violence that is rarely visited upon outsiders, unless they join the dispute at a local event. This feature is one reason why towns are often organized around a single leader or *cacique*, or a group of brothers. Only someone local to the village could understand the issues which drive the conflict, and appropriately adjudicate it. Since legal sanctions are not viable, that person must have the power, or moral persuasion, to enforce solutions.

Religious affiliation

In addition to political identification, religious identification is important in the two communities. While Los Dolores is entirely Catholic, one-quarter of Aqua Fresca's population is Protestant. Conversion to Protestantism has important consequences. In one act, an individual severs himself from all ritual kin ties, and joins a brotherhood of enforced egalitarianism. The individual can be freed from the patterns of patron–client interaction, gift-giving, fiesta sponsorship, and social drinking. At the same time, powerful expectations of eventual economic gain and status mobility are generated. Since religious conversion is often confined to the poorest residents, Protestant identification leads to a paradox of low aggregate wealth for the community, and identification with wealthy 'gringos.'

MULTIPLE HEALTH SYSTEMS: TRADITIONAL AND COSMOPOLITAN MEDICINE

In addition to significant social differences, cultural differences in the perception of illness and its treatment, and in the organization of health systems exist. Clearly, country people are familiar with a large number of practitioners and diseases, and they also believe that many cures are not specific to particular healers. The nurse and spiritists play somewhat intermediate roles. The Auxiliary Nurse is the most frequent contact for country people with MOH services, and often cannot treat many diseases, because of training, logistical and other administrative problems. The spiritist is an extralocal 'traditional' healer, not usually attached to villages.

Diseases also appear to be grouped into categories that predict therapies. Country people do not believe that folk illnesses such as *ojo* or *emphacho* can be cured by cosmopolitan medicine, but the latter also receives low scores in the Aqua Fresca data for *siete dias*, or neonatal tetanus and diabetes. On the other hand, traditional medicine receives low scores for pneumonia, neonatal and infant asphyxiation, typhoid fever, tuberculosis, measles, cancer, and heart disease. Another group of diseases, diarrhoea and dysentery, fevers, worm fever, followed by malnutrition and *flujo*, or flux, can be treated by practically all healers mentioned. VHWs (*parteras*, HGs, and HRs) do not stand out within the traditional medical category, especially in the best implemented site, Aqua Fresca. Country people have a realistic appraisal of their worth. *Parteras* are more highly valued for the treatment of *ojo* and *empacho* than are HGs, and folk healers, such as *sobadoras* and *curanderas* (often treated by informants as a single category), are more highly valued than *parteras*.

A large number of illnesses can be treated at home, and chief among them is the most frequently reported illness, diarrhoea. Since different kinds of healers can cure the same diseases, simultaneous resort can also be anticipated. It should not be imagined that cosmopolitan medicine is considered better for more serious diseases, since *emphaco* and *ojo* are considered two of the most fatal diseases. The patients' own valuation of diseases does not necessarily affect resort to cosmopolitan or folk medicine. Most commonly, country people feel that cosmopolitan medicines are stronger and faster working, but consequently the evaluation of the success of a therapy is more rapid. If cosmopolitan medicines do not resolve the problem in two or three days, patients feel the treatment has failed. Folk remedies are felt to be slower working and are used for chronic disease.

An insight from the questionnaire data (Kendall 1981) is that physicians and hospitals are undifferentiated. Physicians are not separated by service in the MOH, or by work in the clinic or hospital. They are clearly perceived as a distinct profession offering a special kind of therapy, irrespective of locale, but are not seen as promoters of preventive health care. Their services are highly valued for crisis care, and for care that requires hospitalization, but their role is limited. Most interestingly, the overall pattern of response in both communities is very much the same, although Aqua Fresca has been exposed for a much longer time to the VHW programme.

SUCCESS IN AQUA FRESCA

The Health Guardian

The HG in Aqua Fresca does not live in the most central, or the biggest of six hamlets, that make up the town. Her hamlet is closest to the road that leads from Nance to the city, so that she can keep her large store well-stocked with provisions from Nance and the capital. Lori is very successful at all her jobs in the town, and noted for her skill in MOH programmes. She was born in Aqua Fresca, the daughter of the wealthiest man in her hamlet, who was known as a strict diciplinarian, though he taught his children to ride, shoot, and hunt, as well as ensuring that they completed primary school education. This is quite unusual for women in Aqua Fresca, or elsewhere in Nance, and Lori is quite proud of her accomplishments.

After finishing school, Lori married Conejo, also born in Aqua Fresco and from a numerous family, though he was only one of his siblings to attend school, and the only man of his generation in Aqua Fresca to have gone on to study business adminsitration. His own land, and a successful marriage, forms the basis of his current wealth. He is a well-respected man in Aqua Fresca and serves as the local veterinarian, as well as purchasing and selling medicines that he injects himself. His lengthy and varied career outside of

Aqua Fresca has left him with many contacts that he has used to the community's and his own advantage. On his own initiative he found a dentist to visit Aqua Fresca, and approached various private voluntary organizations until he found the funding for Aqua Fresca's piped water system.

Conejo and Lori's current economic conditions reflect their great success in Aqua Fresca. Their store is the only one in town that sells basic grains and sugar. They stock a large range of medicines for sale, in addition to the MOH supplied remedies, which they do not sell. The entire community is, of course, in debt to Conejo and Lori.

Because of their store and other activities, Lori is almost always at home, and attends patients at any hour. She resents leaving her house, but regularly attends the monthly HG sessions in Nance. People visit her most commonly for headaches, coughs and diarrhoea. Lori is a diligent HG and believes in her work. She believes in the germ theory of disease and generally tries to disabuse her neighbours of many folk remedies. On the other hand, she often believes that these folk remedies are efficacious. Although she objects to a number of specific practices, such as the special post-partum diet of dry *tortillas* and cheese, she does follow the healing regimen when she has a cold or sore throat.

Lori claims that she didn't believe in *ojo* until it happened to her own child. Her daughter began vomitting, and although she took the child to the CESAMO and was attended by the physician, the medicines proved ineffective. Finally, in desperation, she took the child to a *sobadora*, who diagnosed it with a fresh egg and prescribed a purgative. The child found practically instant relief, and Lori claims she believes in it still.

A survey conducted in Aqua Fresca demonstrates that country people there value Lori's services. During the previous six months, the 21 households of the sample reported a total of 59 disease episodes. The Ministry programmes are well utilized.

Midwives

A number of other health practitioners are found in Aqua Fresca as well. Among them are the five midwives of the community. Two of the midwives have the midwife kits that are the mark of successful completion of the MOH training programme. They attend the monthly sessions and report the births of the children they help birth. They charge between 10 and 20 Lempiras for their work, depending on the economic conditions of the family. Both of them are elderly women over 60 years of age, and one is a *sobadora*, *curandera*, and bonesetter. Although their participation in the midwife programme formally prohibits their use of medicinal herbs and teas and other traditional birth practices, they do indeed prescribe and use them. They are somewhat reluctant to discuss these practices because they may lose their kits.

Two other midwives who received the course but had to return their kits are famous *curanderas* in the community. The two women are sisters who claim to be 70 and 77 years old. The fact that they do not have their kits does not stop the community from taking advantage of their services, and they deliver many children. Unfortunately though, to avoid a 25 Lempiras fine, they do not report their births to the nurse or to the village HG.

Finally, a fifth midwife is an ancient women, who claims to be over 80 years old, and practises infrequently now. She was, however, the woman who taught most of the other midwives their skills.

There is a great deal of competition among these women for patients, and each one disparages the skills of the other. The MOH kit plays a role in this rivalry, but midwife skills are deemed to be lower than the skills of a good *sobadora* or *curandera*, and all of them make claims for these higher skills.

These health roles are perceived as a calling. They entail onerous obligations and responsibilities, and exposure to dying patients or other disease horrors. Folk healers often resist this calling and only after repeated dreams, or periods of ill health, do they finally take on the curer role. Since the source of this calling is perceived to be supernatural, the supernatural components of the role are deemed to be of higher status than the pragmatic bonesetting or midwifery skills. This is in sharp contrast to recruitment to MOH roles, where very narrow pragmatic tasks define the role, and may perhaps explain why young people are often recruited to these roles, but leave them after a short period.

Community health and success

These observations should demonstrate that the folk medical tradition in Aqua Fresca is very much alive, and that successful practice in this milieu entails modifications to MOH policy. Lori's success as HG in her community would be jeopardized by her rejection of these community expectations. Also, it should not be hard for the reader to imagine that the family derives some real gain from Lori's participation in the VHW programmes, not only from the sale of pharmaceuticals in her store, but also because it is an important community service that she offers for free, precisely because the family has the resources to make it work. Although traditional VHWs are paid, Lori receives the benefit of voluntary service in the goodwill her assistance generates.

That goodwill is necessary, for it is not the case that Lori and Conejo are universally well-liked in their community, and as the single wealthiest family in Aqua Fresca they do attract some resentment. It must not be imagined that Lori and Conejo are good for the MOH, and effective in their communities solely because they have the resources and political power to enforce response. What is also important is that Lori and Conejo are bound, and bind the community, into family and ritual kinship ties, as well as economic and political ones.

Furthermore, the relations between the Protestant minority of Aqua Fresca and the Catholic majority are not always smooth. The HR who makes such a poor showing is co-pastor of the Protestant church in town, and does very little for people who are not his brethren. His selection did not benefit either community organizaton or the health programme. In fact, Conejo effectively serves as HR for the community, but since the Ministry had a policy of not allowing man and wife to serve as HR and HG, he could not formally be named. Nevertheless, when the community does organize under Conejo's leadership, and under the threat of his displeasure, piped water is installed, a school is built, committees are formed, and the community gains the reputation of being progressive.

The success of Aqua Fresca, then, is not so much the success of the MOH programme as the success of Aqua Fresca itself, which is what village-level health programmes are, or should be, about.

FAILURE IN LOS DOLORES

To the encouraging picture of the independently motivated community of Aqua Fresca can be contrasted Los Dolores. The history of MOH contact with Los Dolores is one of frustration on both sides. The initial visit of the Auxiliary Nurse and Promoter had a restrained turnout. When volunteers for the position of HG were requested, no one responded. Older women complained that they could not attend the monthly meetings because of the exigencies of child care. Others hesitated to assume responsibility for the medcines and other equipment the HG was to receive. Finally, a young 17-year-old girl, who had expressed much interest in the clinic and in becoming an Auxiliary Nurse was selected. Within a year of her appointment, she was hired by a nursing supervisor to work as a maid in Tegucigalpa, and pursued her primary education.

The community perceived her selection as a good thing for a large family whose father had deserted them. The daughter had family precedent for the selection, since her mother is a *curandera*, and it is unclear if the mother perceived the selection of her daughter as an opportunity to become a HG without having to attend the monthly sessions personally. This was not, however, the intention of the Auxiliary Nurse, for she did not replace the daughter with her mother. Instead the community remained years without a HG, until July 1981.

The selection of junior persons to fill these voluntary posts continued in the recruitment of the HR. In this case, the eldest son of a recent immigrant to Los Dolores was selected. The son is also a lay Catholic missionary and had an interest in continuing to do good works in the community. Within a year of his appointment, he married and settled in the community. During his tenure, the school latrine was built and three wells dug. His permanence and his commitment to altruistic behaviour were commendable, and at times reinforced the performance of onerous tasks associated with being HR. At other times, however, he felt that his role as HR jeopardized his success as a lay missionary.

The local Health Promoter received from his supervisor goals for construction of latrines. He, in turn, passed these goals on to the local community. To guarantee their construction he attempted to block water projects that the community wanted, but the only latrine constructed in the community was the two-seater found at the school. Although some Los Dolores residents perceive the need for latrines, few if any would consider using one.

Resistance to MOH programmes extends beyond the HG and the HR. The community currently has no *partera* or midwife, let alone a Ministry trained *partera*.

Although it is possible for an *aldea* to depend on nearby *aldeas* to provide the personnel for midwife services, certainly some women in the community must assist at birth. In fact, the word '*partera*' is no longer used in the community, because of its connotations with Ministry training, and the possibility that the man or woman would be held liable by the Health Centre authorities for practising without training. Now there are only birth attendants, and an increasing number of women report that they gave birth to their children alone, or only with assistance of their husbands. In fact, the community is protecting its traditional practitioners. As in many societies, folk medical practice in this community is going 'underground'. Many times, reliance on folk healers or compliance with traditional beliefs are named as causes of resistance to MOH programmes.

The community does organize with the Health Promoter to dig wells, and several families have worked long hours dropping shafts through rock to get at water. However, two of the three wells do not supply water at all in the dry season, and several times during the year the pumps have broken. Furthermore, these wells serve a small proportion of the total population of Los Dolores.

The community also organizes for a number of other projects. The wealthiest man in Los Dolores arranged a 2500 Lempira grant for the construction of a new school. The original schoolhouse was not designed to handle the 110 students and two classrooms, of the current school. The town formed a committee and appointed its wealthiest member as treasurer. He is an older man, and regularly resists appointment as president of committees, although he will actively support their work. He is an accountant by training, and shares a number of other characteristics with Conejo in Aqua Fresca, but he has no store, does not live in the community, and maintains more distant relations with it. In the case of the school project, he simply maintained the books and made disbursements as necessary. Work was subcontracted and the school constructed in record time.

The people of Los Dolores remark that their community does not organize easily, that people who assume responsibility just become targets for slander and abuse. Generally, the persons who can most effectively organize, or assume positions of leadership, are people such as the local wealthy man, who are above reproach, or a patron, or other benefactor of the community. This characteristic is not unexpected given the cultural features previously discussed. It is easy to see that senior exalted persons are better objects of respect than junior equivalent persons, but this is not easy to translate into action, since schooling, wealth, political power, religiosity, family ties, and other factors are all considered when according respect. On the other hand, these individuals may not be as easy to work with as junior people, and their business and other connections may carry them far from their community.

CONCLUSION

The communities of Aqua Fresca and Los Dolores share not only features of climate and topography but also folk medical beliefs and practices, and a host of other social and cultural features. In fact, practically the only attribute they do not share is successful participation in the MOH village level programme. It would be false to conclude that it is only the character of the leading citizens which differs, as this would beg the question of the type of community that generates these arrangements.

Aqua Fresca's leading citizen owns a small store there and was born there. He has much better co-operation in formal activities with the community than his counterpart in Los Dolores. Less social distance separates Conejo and his community than separates the wealthy man of Los Dolores and his community, although in terms of wealth the two men are almost equivalent. Furthermore, Lori was also born in the community, and her job and store bind her daily to it. The wife of Los Dolores' first citizen was not born in town, and she, too, maintains some distance from it.

Aqua Fresca is a community that likes to display a progressive face to the other villages of Nance. The democratic selection of HG worked there because the community knew just whom to select, and the person selected was a mature locally born woman of high social status, whose family had the resources to undertake the job.

On the other hand, the fear of accepting a position of such responsibility in Los Dolores, a community which had never successfully completed a health-oriented project, led to the unsuccessful appointment of two junior community members, one of whom soon left the village. Its local powerful family does not participate as actively in community politics, and its presence marks important class and political divisions within the community.

Clearly, the village contexts are distinctive. The VHW, as member of the MOH team stands between the cosmopolitan and folk medical system, with little or no formal training in medicine. Success in the local community will depend less on learning than on social persona. Thus Ministry programmes will be given a political or religious cast by the persona of the health worker.

Such programmes might work when the leader of the community is selected, but will not be effective if he or she is not. Certainly, one problem is that the HG is perceived as a healer, but is recruited to this role neither in the achieved fashion of cosmopolitan medical training, nor in the traditional fashion of supernatural or family recruitment and training. The role of the HG and the definition of success are far from clear, and numerous other features, both administrative and cultural, complicate the evaluation of the role. Given that the VHW programme continues, what are the social characteristics of the community that promote success?

Just as there are kinds of diseases that country people treat in different ways, there are different kinds of villages and communities. The differences are social and economic, and could be attributed to 'closed' or 'open' community characteristics. Closed and open are not used here in their stricly anthropological sense, where they referred to Indian and Ladino communities respectively, but characterize the way communities respond to community based programmes.

Although there will be varying degrees of openness, a community can be said to be open if it has successfully participated in the past in Ministry or other health-related activities. In this kind of community, the selection of a single HG or HR, and the promotion of culturally appropriate health activities, or the involvement in long-term health education programmes, is likely to have significant benefit.

A closed community, however, is unlikely to respond, at least initially, to this approach. Due to internal strife, high mobility, significant class and power divisions, new programmes become opportunities to redress grievances. Its health personnel are unlikely to participate, respected community members are unlikely to assume positions of responsibility, and its overall level of compliance will be low.

The idea that there are different kinds of communities is certainly not new, but planning for local-level implementation often ignores these community differences, which results in the continued failure of so many VHW Programmes. The problems of VHW desertion and community rejection are not just those of administration and logistics. The cultural distance that separates Ministry health providers from the local rural environment cannot be bridged until health planners develop some respect and understanding for rural laypeople's society and medicine.

References

Achadi, E. and Berman, P. (1988). Growth monitoring in Indonesia: an assessment of coverage and regularity of attendance, Gedangan Village, Central Java, June 1978–November 1981. *United Nations University Food and Nutrition Bulletin*, **10**, 1.

Achard, T. (1983). *Integrated health care in the hills of Nepal*, Integrated Hill Development Project. His Majesty's Government/SATA, Kathmandu, Nepal.

Adams, R. N. (1957). *Cultural survey of Panama—Nicaragua—Guatemala—El Salvador—Honduras*, Pan American Sanitary Bureau Scientific Publication, No. 33. Pan American Sanitary Bureau, Washington, DC.

AFYA (1979). *Inventory of health facilities, 1978*. AFYA Planning Unit, Dar es Salaam.

AFYA (1983). *Guidelines for the implementation of the primary health care programme in Tanzania*. AFYA (Ministry of Health), Dar es Salaam.

AFYA (1989). *Executive summary of the village health workers programme evaluation, 1988*. Mimeo, AFYA, Dar es Salaam.

AFYA/FINIDA/International Development Association (1982). *Village participation in the health workers' training programme*. University of Helsinki Institute of Development Studies, Helsinki.

AFYA/Swedish International Development Authority (1987). *Health centres in need of treatment—a joint evaluation of Sweden's support to the health sector development in Tanzania, 1972–1986*, SIDA Evaluation Report 4 (Health, Tanzania). AFYA/SIDA Dar es Salaam/Stockholm.

Agency for International Development (1977). *Health sector planning*, Project paper, project #522–0148. AID, Honduras.

Alderman, M. H., Husted, J., Levy, B., and Searle, R. (1973). A young-child nutrition programme in rural Jamaica. *Lancet*, **i**, 1166–8.

Allen, S. K. and Goodwin, C. L. (1988). *The KMS chart in Sulawesi, Indonesia: Is growth monitoring working on the periphery of a national expansion?* National Council for International Health, Washington DC.

American Public Health Association (1977). *The state of the art of delivering low cost health services in less developed countries: a summary study of 180 health projects*. APHA, Washington.

Backett, M. (1989). The first forty years: a personal view. *World Health Forum*, **10**, 48–57.

Barbee, E. L. (1986). Biomedical resistance to ethnomedicine in Botswana. *Social Science and Medicine*, **22(1)**, 75–80.

Bastien, J. W. (1990). Community health workers in Bolivia: adapting to traditional roles in the Andean community. *Social Science and Medicine*, **30(3)**, 281–7.

Bennet, F. J. (1981). Community diagnosis: its uses in the training of community health workers and in primary health care in East Africa. *Israel Journal of Medical Sciences*, **17**, 129–37.

Berggren, W. L., Ewbank, D. C., and Berggren, G. G. (1981). Reduction of mortality in rural Haiti through a primary-health-care program. *New England Journal of Medicine*, **304(22)**, 1325–30.

Berman, P. A. (1984). Village health workers in Java, Indonesia: coverage and equity. *Social Science and Medicine*, **19(4)**, 411–22.

Berman, P. A. (1985). *Equity and cost in the organisation of primary health care in Java, Indonesia*, A.E. Research 85–5. Cornell University Department of Agricultural Economics, Ithaca, N. Y.

Berman, P. and Sakai, S. (1992). The productivity of health manpower and supplies in primary health care in rural Java. In *Health economics research in developing countries*, (ed. K. Lee and A. Mills). Oxford University Press. (In press.)

Berman, P., Gwatkin, D. R., and Burger, S. E. (1987). Community-based health workers: head start or false start towards health for all? *Social Science and Medicine*, **25(5)**, 443–59.

Berman, P., Sisler, D. G., and Habicht, J. P. (1989*a*). Equity in public sector primary health care: the role of service organisations in Indonesia. *Economic Development and Cultural Change*, **37(4)**, 777–803.

Berman, P., Brotowasisto, G. O., Mardiati, N., Sakai, S., and Gani, A. (1989*b*). The cost of public primary health care services in rural Indonesia. *Bulletin of the World Health Organization*, **67(6)**, 685–94.

Bibeau, G. (1985). From China to Africa: the same impossible synthesis between traditional and Western medicines. *Social Science and Medicine*, **21(8)**, 937–43.

BIRO Pusat Statisik, Government of Indonesia (1982). *Indikator Kesejahteraan Rakyat (welfare indicators), 1980–81*, Government of Indonesia, Jakarta, Indonesia.

BKKBN, Universities of Udayana, Brawijaya, and Airlangga, Community Systems Foundation (1986). *KB-Gizi—An Indonesian integrated family planning, nutrition, and health program. Final report*. Community Systems Foundation, Ann Arbor, Michigan.

Black, G. (1982). *The triumph of the people*. Zed, London.

Bose, A. (1983). The Community Health Worker scheme: an Indian experiment. In *Practising health for all*, (ed. D. Morley, J. E. Rohde, and G. Williams). Oxford University Press.

Bossert, T. J. and Parker, D. A. (1984). The political and administrative context of primary health care in the Third World. *Social Science and Medicine*, **18(8)**, 693–702.

Braverman, P. A. and Roemer, M. I. (1985). Health personnel training in the Nicaraguan health system. *International Journal of Health Services*, **15**, 699–705.

Brilliant, L., Brilliant, G., Tilden, R., and Pararajasagaram, R. (1985). *The ecology of xerophthalmia in Nepal*. University of Michigan Department of Epidemiology, School of Public Health.

Brotowasisto, G. O., Malik, R., and Sudharto, P. (1988). Health care financing and expenditures in Indonesia. *Health Policy and Planning*, **3(2)**, 131–40.

Bruce-Chwatt, L. J. (1983). Mass drug administration for control of malaria. *Lancet*, **ii**, 688.

Bryant, J. H. (1978). Community health workers: the interface between communities and health care systems. *WHO Chronicle*, **32(4)**, 144–8.

Capps, L. and Crane, P. (1989). Evaluation of a programme to train village health workers in El Salvador. *Health Policy and Planning*, **4(3)**, 239–43.

Carver, R. (1980). The state and popular organisation. *Journal on Social Change and Development*, **8**, 8.

CEDHA (1985). *Ushirikishwaji wa jamii katika mafunzo ya Afya, Mwongozo wautafiti, kitabu cha mafunzo ya Afya*. CEDHA, Arusha.

Center for Nutrition Research and Development (1982). Studi Evaluasi UPGK. In *Penelitian Gizi dan Makanan*. Department of Health, Government of Indonesia, Bogor.

Chagula, W. K. and Tarimo, E. (1975). Meeting basic health needs in Tanzania. In *Health by the people*, (ed. K. W. Newell), pp. 145–68. WHO, Geneva.

Changshu Health Bureau (1986). Consolidation and advance of cooperative medical system in reforms. In *The First conference of the Chinese rural health association*, (ed. Publishing House of China Hospital Administration Journal), pp. 83–87. (Chinese).

Chauls, D. S. and Rajbhandari, P. J. (1980). Nepal's community health leader project. *Rural Development Participation Review*, **11**, 6–8.

Chen, P.-C. and Tuan, C.-H. (1983). Primary health care in rural China: post-1978 development. *Social Science and Medicine*, **17(19)**, 1411–17.

Chen, P. C. Y. and Tan, Y. K. (1981). Primary health care among the Iban of Sarawak. *Tropical and Geographical Medicine*, **33**, 403–9.

Chowdhury, Z. (1981). The good health worker will inevitably become a political figure. *World Health Forum*, **2**, 55–6.

Chung, F. (1988). Education: revolution or reform. In *Zimbabwe's prospects: issues of race, class, state and capital in Southern Africa*, (ed. C. Stoneman), p. 121. Macmillan, London.

Close, D. (1988). *Nicaragua: politics, economics and society*. Pinter, London.

Clyde, D. F. (1962). *History of medical services in Tanganyika*. Government Printer, Dar es Salaam.

Cole-King, S. (1979). *Approaches to the evaluation of maternal and child health care in the context of primary health care*. World Health Organization, HSM/79.2, Geneva.

Cole-King, S. Gordon, G., and Lovell, H. (1979). Evaluation of primary health care—a case study of Ghana's rural health care system. *Journal of Tropical Medicine and Hygiene*, November/December, 214–28.

Comision Popular Salud Region Zona Especial II (1984). *Abriendo La trocha Brigadistas defienden salud y la revolucion en Zelaya Sur*. Primer Congreso Nacional Journadas Populares de Salud, Managua.

Conlin, S. and Falk, A. (1979). *Kosi Hill area rural development programme (KHARDEP), Nepal: a study of the socioeconomy of the Kosi Hill area. Guidelines for planning an integrated rural development programme*. Vol. 1, KHARDEP Report No. 3. Overseas Development Agency/Land Resources Development Centre, Nepal.

Consejo Nacional Popular de Salud (1984). *La participación de las organiziciones populares en la gestion de salud*. Primer Congreso Nacional Jornadas Populares de Salud, Managua.

Coordinación Nacional de las Jornadas Populares de Salud (1984). *Las Jornadas populares de salud en sus tres anos de desarrollo*. CNJPS, Managua.

Coyle, E. F. (1984). *Health Services in Zelaya Sur: Special Zone II. Report*. Catholic Institute for International Relations, London.

Dave, J. (1960). *Ten-point programme of rural welfare*. Navjivan Publishing House, Ahmedabad.

De Kadt, E. (1983). Community participation for health: the case of Latin America. In *Practising health for all*, (ed. D. Morley, J. E. Rohde, and G. Williams). Oxford University Press.

Deodhar, N. S. (1986). Main gaps and constraints in our approach to and programmes for provision of primary health care. In *Health for all: concept and reality*, (ed. S. Gill). Foundation for Research in Community Health, Bombay.

Department of Health, Direktorat Bina Upaya Kesehatan PusKesMas, BKKBN, Lembaga Demografi Universitas Indonesia, Fakultas Kesehatan Masyarakat Universitas Indonesia, US. Agency for International

Development (1988). *Laboran Studi Analisis Pembiayaan Pos Yandu di Indonesia. (Report of the Indonesia Pos Yandu cost study)*. Mimeo. Department of Health, Jakarta, Indonesia.

Department of Medical Adminstration (DMA), Ministry of Public Health (1986). *A national sample survey of rural health services*. Unpublished. MOPH, Beijing. (Chinese).

Direccion General de Estadisticas y Censos (1980). *Anuario Estadistico, 1978*. Ministerio de Economia, Tegucigalpa, Honduras.

Donahue, J. M. (1986). *The Nicaragua revolution in health*. Bergin and Garvey, Massachussetts.

Draft Sixth Five Year Plan (1979). *Draft sixth five year plan, 1979–83 (revised)*. Planning Commission, New Delhi.

Ebrahim, G. J. (1962). A model of integrated community health care. *Tropical and Geographical Medicine*, **28**, S5–S52.

Eggan, F. (1954). Social anthropology and the method of controlled comparison. *American Anthropologist*, **56**, 743–63.

Ellesberg, M. (1982). Educacion y participacion popular en salud. *Revista Centro Americana de Ciencia de la Salud*, **23**, 145–61.

England, R. (1978). More myths in international health planning. *American Journal of Public Health*, **68(2)**, 153–59.

Eoff, G. (1980). *Vista socio-cultural de la salud rural y la entrega de servicios de salud: mito y realidad*, Informe No. 4, AID/552–T–490. US. Agency for International Development, Tegucigalpa, Honduras.

Eshuis, J. (1980). *Medical auxiliary training in Tanzania: relevance for the realisation of integrated primary health care*. Dissertation for the 16th International Course in Health Development, 1979–1980, Prinz Leopold Institute, Antwerp.

Essex, B. (1980). A new approach to decision making in primary health care. *Proceedings of the Royal Society of London*, **B 209**, 89–96.

Evaluation and Planning Cente (EPC), London School of Hygiene and Tropical Medicine (1988). *Health promoters in Colombia: is preventive care sufficient?* In *Community health workers: policy and practice in national programmes* (ed. G. Walt). London School of Hygiene and Tropical Medicine, Evaluation and Planning Centre.

Fajans, P. and Sudiman, H. (1983). *The Indonesian national family planning improvement program: a case study of seven villages*. Mimeo. United Nations International Children's Emergency Fund, Jakarta.

Fals-Borda, O. (1987). The application of participatory action-research in Latin America. *International Sociology*, **2**, 329–47.

Fendall, N. R. E. (1972). Forerunners. *World Health Magazine*, **2**, 4–7.

Fendall, N. R. E. and Tiwari, I. C. (1980). Trends in primary health care. *Tropical Doctor*, **10**, 78–85.

Fewer, D. J. (1982). *Encuesta Demográphica Nacional de Nicaragua. Analysis de los preguntas retrospectivas*. CELADE, San Jose.

Flahault, D. (1978). The relationship between community health workers, the health services, and the community. *WHO Chronicle*, **32**, 149–53.

Foote D. L., Hughes-Lind, L., Kendall, C., Martorell, R., McDivitt, J. A., Snyder, L., Stome, S. M., and Storey, J. D. (1985). *The mass media and health practices evaluation in Honduras: findings from the first two years*. Applied Communication Technology, Menlo Park, CA.

Ford Foundation (1987). *Amubhav: experiments in community health*. (Series of 12 publications: Streehitkarini; KEM Rural Health Project; Banwasi Seva Ashram; Comprehensive Health and Development Project, Pachod; Child In Need Institute; Comprehensive Labour Welfare Scheme of United Planters Associasion of Southern India (UPASI); Rural Unit for Health and Social Affairs; Mini Health Centre Programme of VHS; Community-based Contraceptive Distribition Programme of Family Planning Association of India (FPAI) and BHU; Action for Welfare and Awakening in Rural Environment; Society for Education, Welfare and Action-Rural; Parivar Seva Sanstha.) Rural Unit of Health and Social Affairs, New Delhi.

Ford Foundation (1988). *Action for welfare and awakening in rural environment* Ford Foundation, New Delhi.

Frank, J. W. (1981). *Primary health care systems utilising auxiliaries: problems and prospects in the 1980s with special reference to Tanzania*. Unpublished Master of Science dissertation, London School of Hygiene and Tropical Medicine.

Frankel, S. J. (1982). *Family health services and the organisation of health care in Tari*. Southern Highlands Provincial Government, Mendi, Papua New Guinea.

Frankel, S. J. (1984). Peripheral health workers are central to primary health care: lessons from Papua New Guinea's aid posts. *Social Science and Medicine*, **19(3)**, 279–90.

Frankel, S. J. (1986). *The Huli response to illness*. Cambridge University Press.

Frankel, S. J. and Lehmann, D. (1984). Oral rehydration therapy: combining epidemiological and anthropological approaches in the evaluation of a Papua New Guinea programme. *Journal of Tropical Medicine and Hygiene*, **87**, 137–42.

Frankel, S. J. and Lewis, G. (1989). *A continuing trial of treatment: medical pluralism in Papua New Guinea*, Kluwer, Dortrecht.

Frankenberg, E. (1987). *Direct costs of the Pos Yandu: a model for analysis*. Mimeo prepared for United States Agency for International Development, Jakarta.

Frieden, T. and Garfield, R. (1987). Popular participation in health in Nicaragua. *Health Policy and Planning*, **2**, 162–70.

Fu, D. W. *et al*. (1987). Exploration of multiple forms of village health care units. In *Health policies and administration*, (ed. Expert Committee on Health Policy and Administration), pp. 58–69. MOPH, Beijing. (Chinese).

Gandhi, M. K. (1945). *Constructive programme: its meaning and place*. Navjivan Publishing House, Ahmedabad.

Gao, N.S. (1987). Today's Shanghai county. *Acta Academiae Medicinae Shanghai*. Supplement 1–4, (Chinese).

Garfield, R. M. (1989). War related changes in health and health services in Nicaragua. *Social Science and Medicine*, **28(7)**, 669–76.

Garfield, R. M. and Rodriguez, P. F. (1985). Health and health services in Central America. *JAMA*, **254**, 936–43.

Garfield, R. M. and Vermund, S. H. (1983). Changes in Malaria incidence after mass drug administration in Nicaragua. *Lancet*, **i**, 500–3.

Garfield, R. M. and Vermund, S. H. (1986). Health education and community participation in mass drug administration for malaria in Nicaragua. *Social Science and Medicine*, **22**, 869–77.

Garfield, R. M. and Williams, G. (1989). *Health and revolution: the Nicaraguan experience*. OXFAM, Oxford.

Garfield, R. M., Prado, E., Gates, J. R., and Vermund, S. H. (1989). Malaria in Nicaragua: community-based control efforts and the impact of the war. *International Journal of Epidemiology*, **18**, 434–9.

Gilmurray, J., Riddell, R., and Sanders, D. (1979). *The struggle for health*. Catholic Institute for International Relations, London.

Gish, O. (1973). Doctors auxiliaries in Tanzania. *Lancet*, **ii**, 1251–4.

Gish, O. (1975). Village and mobile services. In *Planning the health sector: The Tanzanian experience*. (ed. O. Gish), pp. 128–9. Croom Helm, London.

Goitre and Cretinism Eradication Project (GCEP) (1987). *Iodine deficiency disorders in Nepal: assessment of programme impact and future strategy*. GCEP, Kathmandu, Nepal.

Gong, Y. L. (1986). *Needs of medical services*. Shanghai Medical University, Shanghai, (Chinese).

Gong, Y. L. and Chao, L. M. (1982). The role of barefoot doctors. *American Journal of Public Health*, **72(9)**, Supplement 59–61.

Gonzalez, M. (1990). *Nicaragua: what went wrong?* Bookmarks, London.

Government of Indonesia and United Nations International Children's Emergency Fund (1988). *Annual Review: Review of REPELITA. IV: Cooperation in Nutrition*. Unpublished manuscript. Government of Indonesia, Jakarta.

Groman, P. and McConnell, C. (1978). *Village health worker training programme: preliminary report*. Mimeo. Britain Nepal Medical Trust, Biratnagar, Nepal.

Habicht, J-P. (1982). Learning from failure. *World Health Forum*, **3(1)**, 81–2.

Haliman, A. and Williams, G. (1983). Can people move bureaucratic mountains? Developing primary health care in rural Indonesia. *Social Science and Medicine*, **17(19)**, 1449–55.

Haraldson, S. S. R. (1988). Community health aides for sparse populations. *World Health Forum*, **9**, 235–8.

Harrison, P. (1981). Success story. *World Health*, Feb–March, 14–19.

He, Q. Y. *et al*. (1987). Exploration of health care system reforms in Liaozhong county. *China Public Health (Management Edition)*, **3(1)**, 27–9. (Chinese).

Heggenhougen, H. K. (1984). Will primary care efforts be allowed to succeed? *Social Science and Medicine*, 19, 217–24.

Heggenhougen, H. K. (1986). Health services: official and unofficial. In *Tanzania, crisis and struggle for survivial*, (ed. J. Boesen, J. Havnevik, J. Koponene, and R. Odgaard), Scandinavian Institute of African Studies, Uppsala.

Heggenhougen, H. K. and Mkumbwa, Z. M. (1982). Village health workers for primary health care in Tanzania. *Nordisk Medicine*, **97**, 61–2.

Heggenhougen, H. K., Vaughan, P., Mohondwa, E. P. Y., and Rutabanzibwa-Ngaiza, J. (1987). *Community health workers: the Tanzanian experience*. Oxford University Press.

Heiby, J. R. (1982). Some lessons from Nicaragua. *World Health Forum*, **3(1)**, 27–9.

His Majesty's Government National Planning Commission (1987). *Programme for fulfilment of basic needs (1985–2000)*. Singha Durbar, Kathmandu, Nepal.

His Majesty's Government Nepal (1975). *Nepal nutrition status survey*. United States Agency for International Development Office of Nutrition, Washington, DC.

His Majesty's Government Nepal (1982). *Report of workshop on strengthening community participation in health through the Community Health Leader Program*. Ministry of Health, Kathmandu, Nepal.

His Majesty's Government Nepal (1988). *Country health profile*. HMG, Kathmandu, Nepal.

Hopkinson, A. and Chalmers, F. (1990). Nicaragua: the first 100 days. *Lancet*, **336**, 300–1.

Huaiyou Health Bureau (1986). Consolidation of three-layer health care network. In *The First Conference of the Chinese Rural Health Association*, (ed. Publishing House of China Hospital Administration Journal), pp. 39–41. (Chinese).

Huang, S. M. (1988). Transforming China's collective health care system: a village study. *Social Science and Medicine*, **27(9)**, 879–88.

Indian Council of Medical Research (ICMR)-Indian Council of Social Science Research (ICSSR) (1981). *Health for all—an alternative strategy*. Indian Institute of Education, Pune.

Instituto Nacional de Estadisticas y Cenos (INEC)-Centro Latinoamericano de Demografía, (CELADE) Nicaragua (1983). Estimaciones y proyecciones de poblacion; 1950–2025. Fasciculo F-NIC 1. In *Cambridge encyclopaedia of Latin America and the Caribbean*, (ed. S. Collier, H. Blackmore, and J. Skidmore). Cambridge University Press.

Islam, K. and Bachman, S. (1983). Primary Health Care in Bangladesh—too much to ask? *Social Science and Medicine*, **17(19)**, 1463–66.

Jacobson, M., Becerra, F., Labbok, M., Parker, R., and Akinyi, J. (1987). Time distribution of CHW activities: does curative care preclude preventive care? *Health Policy and Planning*, **2(1)**, 85–9.

Janzen, J. M. (1978). *The quest for therapy in Lower Zaire*. University of California Press.

Jobert, B. (1985). Populism and health policy: the case of community health volunteers in India. *Social Science and Medicine*, **20(1)**, 1–28.

Johnston, M. (1983). The ant and the elephant: voluntary agencies and government health programs in Indonesia. In *Practising health for all*, (ed. D. Morley, J. E. Rohde, and G. Williams), pp. 168–89. Oxford University Press.

Joint Secretary of the Union Ministry of Health and Family Welfare (1981). *Communication of the scheme to Health Secretaries of States and Union Territories*, D.O. No P.18014/4/80-RHD. Ministry of Health and Family Welfare, New Delhi.

Judd, M. (1987). *Village kader study: an investigation of kaders in five West Java villages*. Mimeo. USAID, Indonesia.

Justice, J. (1983). The invisible worker: the role of the peon in Nepal's health service. *Social Science and Medicine*, **17(14)**, 967–70.

Kendall, C. (1981). *An enthnographic evaulation of the Honduran Village Health Worker program: a controlled comparison of two villages*. Project No. P-47–81, Integrated Rural Health. USAID, Tegucigalpa, Honduras.

Kendall, C. (1983). Loose structure of family in Honduras. *Journal of Comparative Family Studies*, **14(2)**, 257–72.

Kendall, C. (1984). Ethnomedicine and oral rehydration therapy: a case study of ethnomedical investigation and program planning. *Social Science and Medicine*, **19(3)**, 253–60.

Kielmann, A. A., Taylor, C. E., and Parker, R. L. (1978). The Narangwal nutrition study: a summary review. *American Journal of Clinical Nutrition*, **31**, 2040–52.

King, M. (ed.) (1966). *Medical care in developing countries*. Oxford University Press.

Kleinman, A. (1980). *Patients and healers in the context of culture*. University of California Press.

Lamboray, J.-L. and Laing, C. (1984). Partners for better health. *World Health Forum*, **5**, 30–4.

Lamptey, P. R., Nicholas, D. D., and Quartey-Papafio, E. (1980). Training village health workers in rural Ghana. *World Health Forum*, **1(1/2)**, 52–6.

Lane, R. A. (1981). Tanzania: medicine on a meagre budget. *Canadian Medical Association Journal*, **124**, 506–13.

Lenin, V. I. (1976). The state and revolution. In *Selected works*, Vol. 2. Progress Publishers, Moscow.

Leslie, C. (1976). The ambiguities of medical revivalism in modern India. In *Asian medical system*, (ed. C. Leslie), pp. 356–67. University of California Press.

Loewenson, R. (1985). *Social services in rural council areas*, Ministry of Health Mimeo. Save the Children Fund (UK), Harare.

Loewenson, R. and Sanders, D. (1988). Political economy of health and nutrition. In *Zimbabwe's prospects: issues of race, class, state and capital in Southern Africa* (ed. C. Stoneman). Macmillan, London.

McCord, C. and Kielmann, A. A. (1978). A successful programme for medical auxiliaries treating childhood diarrhoea and pneumonia. *Tropical Doctor*, **8**, 220–25.

Magari, F. M. and Kikoito, N. I. (1983). *Organisation and implementation of primary health care in Tanzania*. In *Community health workers*, report of the interregional study and workshop, 4–8 July 1983, SHS/HMD/84.1. WHO, Geneva.

Mandel, E. (1978). *From Stalinism to Eurocommunism*. NLB, London.

Mangelsdorf, K. R. (1988). The selection and training of primary health care workers in Ecuador: issues and alternatives for public policy. *International Journal of the Health Servies*, **18(3)**, 471–93.

Manoff International (1984). *Nutrition communication and behaviour change component: Indonesian Nutrition Development Program Project Description*. Manoff International, New York.

Marchione, T. J. (1984). Evaluating primary health care and nutrition programs in the context of national development. *Social Science and Medicine*, **19(3)**, 225–35.

Maru, R. M. (1983). The community health volunteer scheme in India: an evaluation. *Social Science and Medicine*, **17(19)**, 1477–83.

Matomora, M. K. S. (1989). Mass produced village health workers and the promise of primary health care. *Social Science and Medicine*, **28(10)**, 1081–4.

Mattaka, D. (1977). *The problems of training medical auxiliaries in Tanzania*. Unpublished dissertation for the Diploma in Tropical Public Health, London School of Hygiene and Tropical Medicine.

Mburu, F. M. and Boerma, J. T. (1989). Community-based health care 10 years post Alma Ata. *Social Science and Medicine*, **28(10)**, 1005–6.

Miller, V. (1985). *Between struggle and hope: the Nicaraguan literacy crusade*. Westview Press, Boulder.

Ministry of Community and Co-operative Development (1989). *Village Community Workers*. Mimeo press release 24/2/89. MCCD, Harare.

Ministry of Community and Co-operative Development and Women's Affairs (1988). *Report on seminars to plan for village community worker training*. Mimeo, MCCD. Harare.

Ministry of Community and Co-operative Development and Women's Affairs (1989). *The Village Community Worker Training Programme*. National Consultative Workshop for Provincial Training Teams, Kadoma Ranch Motel. MCCD, Harare.

Ministry of Health (1982). *Report on the Village Health Worker Evaluation Project*. Government of Zimbabwe, Harare.

Ministry of Health (1983*a*). *Report of the National Health Manpower Planning and Projections Workshop*. Government of Zimbabwe, Harare.

Ministry of Health (1983*b*). *Evaluation of the Village Health Workers Programme*. Government of Zimbabwe, Harare.

Ministry of Health (1984*a*). *Planning for equity in health*. Government of Zimbabwe, Harare.

Ministry of Health (1984*b*). *Report on a joint mission to evaluate primary health care in Zimbabwe*. Government of Zimbabwe, Harare.

Ministry of Health (1984*c*). *Zimbabwe Primary Health Care Review*, **1**, 5.

Ministry of Public Health (1984). *Chinese health year book*. People's Health Publishing House, Beijing. (Chinese).

Ministry of Public Health (1985). *Chinese health year book*. People's Health Publishing House. Beijing. (Chinese).

Ministry of Public Health (1987). *Chinese health statistical digest*. MOPH, Beijing. (Chinese).

MINSA (Ministerio de Salud, Nicaragua) (1980). *¿Qué es el sistema nacional de salud?* Boletin, 1. MINSA, Managua.

MINSA (Ministerio de Salud, Nicaragua) (1982*a*). *Programma Integral de Activades del Area de Salud (PIAAS)*. Libro Rojo Y Negro. MINSA, Managua.

MINSA (Minsterio de Salud, Nicaragua) (1982*b*). *Sanemiento ambiental. Jornada Popular de Salud*. MINSA, Managua.

MINSA (Ministerio de Salud, Nicaragua) (1983). *Plan Nacional de Salud, 1984*. MINSA, Managua.

MINSA (Ministerio de Salud, Nicaragua) (1987). *Plan de Salud, 1988–1990*. MINSA, Managua.

MINVAH (Ministerio de Viviendas y Asentamientos Humanos, Nicaragua) (1987*a*). *Estatísticas*. MINVAH, Managua.

MINVAH (Ministerio de Viviendas y Asentamientos Humanos, Nicaragua) (1987*b*). *Sistema de asentamientos de Zona Especial II y Esquema Urbano de La Cuidad de Bluefields*. MINVAH Managua.

Mkumbwa, Z. M. (1978). *The training of village health workers in the context of villagisation in Tanzania: a project report*. WHO Regional Teacher Training Centre, University of New South Wales, Kensington, Australia.

Mkumbwa, Z. M. (1983). *Kitabu cha mafunzo ya mhudumu wa afya kijijini*. Benedictine Publications, Ndanda-Peramino, Tanzania.

Morley, D. (1973). *Paediatric priorities in the developing world*. Butterworths, London.

Morley, D., Rohde, J. E., and Williams, G. (ed.) (1983). *Practising health for all*. Oxford University Press.

Mtey, P. J. B. (1977). *Towards health by the people*. Unpublished dissertation for the Diploma in Tropical Public Health, London School of Hygiene and Tropical Medicine.

Muhondwa, E. P. Y. (1982). *Population participation in health care: a study of the factors underlying the acceptability of, and participation in, three health care programmes by rural populations in Tanga, Tanzania*. Unpublished Ph.D. thesis, University of Nottingham.

Mukhopadhyay, M. (1983). Human development through primary health care: case studies from India. In *Practising health for all*, (ed. D. Morley, J. E. Rohde, and G. Williams). Oxford University Press.

Mwambulambo, D. J. (1977). *The village health workers scheme in Tanzania*. Unpublished paper to the Airlie House Conference, Oct 26–28, International Medical Research Foundation, New York.

Nabarro, D., Cassels, C., Pant, M., and Wijga, A. (1987). *The impact of integrated rural development: the Kosi Hill area rural development programme, East Nepal*, Department of International Community Health, Liverpool, UK.

Nabarro, D., Pant, M., Cassels, C., Wijga, A., Howard, P., and Padfield, N. (1988). The importance of infectious and environmental factors as possible determinants of growth retardation in children. In *Linear growth retardation in less developed countries*, (ed. J.C. Waterlow), Nestle Nutrition Workshop Series, Volume 14. Raven Press, New York.

Nabarro, D., Cassels, C., and Pant, M. (1989). How households cope in the hills of Nepal: can development initiatives help? *IDS Bulletin*, **20(2)** 68–74.

National Planning Committee (1948). *Report of the sub-committee on health*. NPC, New Delhi.

Nepal Planning Commission (1979). *Basic principles of the Sixth Plan (1980–1985)*. HMG, Kathmandu, Nepal.

New Era (1986). *A baseline survey for the Joint Nutrition Support Programme*. New Era, Kathmandu, Nepal.

Newell, K. (ed.) (1975). *Health by the people*. World Health Organization, Geneva.

Nove, A. (1983). *The economics of feasible socialism*. Allen and Unwin, London.

Nyerere, J. K. (1968). Ujamaa, the basis of African socialism; The Arusha Declaration; Socialism and rural development. In *Ujamaa essays on socialism*, pp. 1–12, 13–37, 107–44. Oxford University Press.

Nyerere, J. K. (1977). *The Arusha Declaration ten years after*. Government Printer, Dar es Salaam.

Ofosu-Amaah, V. (1983). *National experience in the use of community health workers: a review of current issues and problems*, Offset Publication No. 71. WHO, Geneva.

Paul, B. D. (1958). The role of beliefs and customs in sanitation programs. *American Journal of Public Health*, **48**, 1502–6.

Political Bureau of the Chinese Communist Party Central Committee (PBCCPCC) (1987). Several points in current rural economic policies. In *Persist in reforms, opening and activities*, (ed. SCCPCC). People's Publishing House, Beijing.

Radford, A. J. (1978). Village-based health and medical care resources. In *Basic health care in developing countries: an epidemiological perspective*, (ed. B. Hetzel), pp. 146–69. Oxford University Press.

Ramprasad, A. (1988). Community health workers—an evolving force. *World Health Forum*, **9**, 229–34.

Reid, R. A., Ruffing, K. L., and Smith H. L. (1986). Managing medical supply logistics among health workers in Ecuador. *Social Science and Medicine*, **22(1)**, 9–14.

Rifkin, S. B. (1980). Health care in China: the experts take command. *Tropical Doctor*, **10**, 86–90.

Rifkin, S. B. (1983). Primary health care in Southeast Asia: attitudes about community participation in community health programmes. *Social Science and Medicine*, **17(19)**, 1489–96.

Rohde, J. E. (1983). Health for all in China: principles and relevance for other countries. In *Practising health for all*, (ed. D. Morley, J.E. Rohde, and G. Williams), pp. 5–16. Oxford University Press.

Rohde, J. E. and Hendrata, L. (1983). Development from below: transformation from village-based nutrition projects to a national family nutrition program in Indonesia. In *Practising health for all*, (ed. D Morley, J.E Rohde, and G. Williams), pp. 252–71. Oxford University Press.

Rohde J. E. and Northrup, R. S. (1977). *Mother as the basic health worker: training her and her trainers*. Paper presented at Bellagio Consultation on the New Type of Basic Health Service World-Wide and the Implications for the Education of Other Health Care Professionals.

Ronaghy, H. A. and Solter, S. (1974). Is the Chinese 'barefoot doctor' exportable to rural Iran? *Lancet*, **i**, 1331–3.

Rubel, A. (1964). The epidemiology of a folk illness: Susto in Hispanic America. *Ethnology*, **3**, 268–83.

Ruchwarger, G. (1985). The Sandinista mass organisations and the revolutionary process. In *Nicaragua: a revolution under siege*, (ed. R. Harris and C. Vilas). Zed, London.

Sanders, D. (1980). *Some guideline proposals for a national village health worker scheme in Zimbabwe*. Unpublished mimeo.

Sanders, D. (1984). The state and popular organisation. *Journal on Social Change and Development*, **8**, 6–8.

Sanders, D. (1985). *The struggle for health*. Macmillan, London.

Sanders, D. and Davies, R. (1988). Economic adjustment and current trends in child survival: the case of Zimbabwe. *Health Policy and Planning*, **3(3)**, 198.

Scholl, E. A. (1985). An assessment of community health workers in Nicaragua. *Social Science and Medicine*, **20(3)**, 207–14.

Schulpen, T. W. J. (1975). *Integration of church and government medical services in Tanzania—effects at district level*. AM-REF, Nairobi.

Segal, M. (1973). The politics of health in Tanzania. *Development and Change*, **4**, 39–50.

Shah, U., Pratinidhi, A. K. Bhatlawande, P. V., and Alekar, S. V. (1984). Using community health workers to screen for anaemia. *World Health Forum*, **5**, 35–6.

Shearly, A. E. (1988). *A study on how the changed role of the village community workers has affected primary health care at primary level*. Research project for Diploma in Nursing Administration, Harare.

Shi, Y. S. (1986). Direction of rural medical service system under the new situation. *Chinese Rural Health Service Administration*, **4–5**, 47–51. (Chinese).

Shong, J. X. (1988). Analyses for reasons of closing down 168 village health stations. *Chinese Rural Health Service Administration*, **4**, 31–3.

Sidel, V. and Sidel, R. (1974). *Serve the people: observations on medicine in the People's Republic of China*, Beacon Press, Boston.

Signer, E. and Galston, A. W. (1972). Education and science in China. *Science*, **175**, 15–23.

Smyly, P. A. J. (1988). *OXFAM primary health care project in Manicaland province, Zimbabwe: 6th report and progress review*. Elim Hospital, Nyanga.

Stark, R. (1985). Lay workers in primary health care: victims in the process of social transformation. *Social Science and Medicine*, **20(3)**, 269–75.

State Statistical Bureau (1987). *Chinese statistical year book*. Chinese Statistical Publishing House, Beijing. (Chinese).

State Statistical Bureau (1988). *A statistical survey of China*. Chinese Statistical Publishing House, Beijing, (Chinese).

Stone, L. (1986). Primary health care for whom? Village perspectives from Nepal. *Social Science and Medicine*, **22(3)**, 293–302.

Storms, D. M. (1979). *Training and use of auxiliary health workers: lessons from developing countries*, American Public Health Association. International Health Programs Monograph Series, No. 3. APHA, Washington, DC.

Suyadi, A., Sadjimin, T. and Rohde, J. E. (1977). Primary care in the village: an approach to village self-help health programs. *Tropical Doctor*, July, 123–8.

Tarimo, E. (1978). Health and self-reliance: the experience of Tanzania. *Development Dialogue*, **1**, 35–40.

Tarimo, E. and Fowkes, F. G. R. (1989). Strengthening the backbone of primary health care. *World Health Forum*, **10**, 74–9.

Taylor, M., Shresthra, R. B., Rajbhandari, P., and Shresthra, M. (1989). *Community health volunteer program: orientations and first phase training review*. John Snow Inc., Kathmandu, Nepal.

Taylor, P. (1988). *Community health volunteers: program review and recommendations*. Public Health Division, Ministry of Health/United States Agency for International Development, Kathmandu, Nepal.

Tesh, S. (1986). Health education in Cuba: a preface. *International Journal of Health Services*, **16**, 87–104.

Thomas, I. D. (1983). *Population and health facilities in Tanzania–1978*, Regional Atlas for Mainland Rural Regions, Vol. 3. University of East Anglia, Overseas Development Group, Norwich.

Thompson, N. (1984). Australian aboriginal health and health-care. *Social Science and Medicine*, **18(11)**, 939–48.

Titmuss, R. M., Abel-Smith, B., Macdonald, G., Williams, A. W. and Wood, C. H. (1964). *The health services of Tanganyika—a report to the government*. Pitman, London.

Tucker, M. (1989). Nicaragua: ten years after the revolution. *Social Organiser*, **17**, 412–13.

Tumwine, J. (1988). *OXFAM primary health care project in Manicaland province, Zimbabwe: a report of the first 4 years in Chimanimani district (Dec 83–Dec 87)*. OXFAM, Zimbabwe.

Tumwine, J. K. (1989) Community participation as myth or reality: a personal experience from Zimbabwe. *Health Policy and Planning*, **4(2)**, 157–61.

Turshen, M. (1984). *The political ecology of disease in Tanzania*. Rutgers University Press, New Brunswick.

Twumasi, P. A. and Freund, P. J. (1985). Local politicization of primary health care as an instrument for development: a case study of community health workers in Zambia. *Social Science and Medicine*, **20(10)**, 1073–80.

Ugalde, A. (1985). Ideological dimensions of community participation in Latin American health programs. *Social Science and Medicine*, **21**, 41–53.

United Nations International Childrens Emergency Fund (1986). *From child growth monitoring towards integrated delivery of child survival and development services: the Indonesian experience*. UNICEF, Jakarta.

United Nations International Childrens Emergency Fund (1987). *Children and women of Nepal: a situation analysis*. UNICEF, Kathmandu, Nepal.

United Nations International Childrens Emergency Fund/World Health Organization (1980). *Primary health care: the community health worker*. Report on an Interregional Study and Workshop (Kingston, Jamaica), PHC/80.2. World Health Organization, Geneva.

Van Etten, G. M. (1971). New strategies of rural health development. *Tropical and Geographical Medicine*, **23**, 393–8.

Van Etten, G. M. (1976). *Rural health development in Tanzania—a case study of medical sociology in a developing country*. Van Gorcum & Co., Assen.

Vaughan, J. P. and Walt, G. (1983). Village health workers and primary health care. *Tropical Doctor*, **13**, 105–8.

Veraguas, S. (1982). *Report on 'parteras' (traditional birth attendants) in Region I of Nicaragua*. Catholic Institute for International Relations, London.

Villegas, H. (1977). Extension of health service coverage in Costa Rica. *Bulletin of the Pan American Health Organization*, **9(4)**, 303–10.

Waloeyo Cokrodarmanto (1976). *Pembangunan Kesehatan Masyarakat Desi di Kabupaten Daerah Tinkat II Karanganyar*. Paper presented at the National Primary Health Care Seminar, Jakarta.

Walt, G. (1988*a*). CHWs: are national programmes in crisis? *Health Policy and Planning*, **3(1)**, 1–21.

Walt, G. (1988*b*). *Community health workers: policy and practice in national programmes*. Publication No. 16. London School of Hygiene and Tropical Medicine, Evaluation and Planning Centre.

Walt, G. (ed.) (1990). *Community health workers in national programmes: just another pair of hands?* Open University Press, Milton Keynes.

Walt, G., Ross, D., Gilson, L., Owuor-Omondi, L., and Knudsen, T. (1989). Community health workers in national programmes: the case of the family welfare educators of Botswana. *Transactions of the Royal Society of Tropical Medicine and Hygiene*, **83**, 49–55.

Wang, V. L. (1975). Training of the barefoot doctor in the People's Republic of China: from prevention to curative service. *International Journal of Health Services*, **5**, 475–88.

Wang, Y. M. and Deng, W. (1988). A survey on the professional quality and training of VHWs. *Chinese Rural Health Service Administration*, **7**, 45–8. (Chinese).

Weed, L. L. (1968). Medical records that teach and guide. *New England Journal of Medicine*, **278(11)**, 652–7.

Wellin, E. (1955). Water boiling in a Peruvian town. In *Healing, culture and community*, (ed. B. Paul). Russel Sage, New York.

Werner, D. (1977). *Where there is no doctor*. The Hesperian Foundation, Palo Alto.

Werner, D. (1981). The village health worker—lackey or liberator. *World Health Forum*, **2(1)**, 46–54.

Werner, D. (1983). Health care in Cuba: a model service or a means of social control—or both? In *Practising health for all*, (ed. D. Morley, J.E. Rohde, and G. Williams). Oxford University Press.

Werner, D. and Bower, B. (1982). *Helping health workers learn*. The Hesperian Foundation, Palo Alto.

White G. (1983). Introduction. In *Revolutionary socialist development in the Third World*, (G. White, R. Murray, and C. White). Harvester Press, Guildford, Surrey.

Williams, G. (1988). WHO—the days of mass campaigns. *World Health Forum*, **9**, 7–23.

Williams, G. and Satoto (1983). Socio-political constraints on primary health care. In *Practising health for all*, (ed. D. Morley, J. E. Rohde, and G. Williams), pp. 208–228. Oxford University Press.

Wilson, P. A. (1987). Regionalisation and decentralisation in Nicaragua. *Latin American Perpectives*, **14(2)**, 237–54.

World Bank (1979). *Nepal: development performance and prospects*. World Bank, South Asia Regional Office.

World Health Organization (1978*a*). *Primary health care*. Report of the International Conference on Primary Health Care, Alma-Ata, USSR, 6–12 September 1978. World Health Organization, Geneva.

World Health Organization (1978*b*). *Lay reporting of health information*. World Health Organization, Geneva.

World Health Organization (1980). *The primary health worker*. World Health Organization, Geneva.

World Health Organization (1984). *Community health workers*, Report of the Inter-Regional Study and Workshop, 4–8 July 1983, SHS/HMD/84.1. WHO, Geneva.

World Health Organization (1986*a*). *Report of interregional planning meeting on strengthening the performance of community health workers in primary health care, New Delhi 2–4 December 1985*. World Health Organization, Geneva.

World Health Organization (1986*b*). *Weekly Epidemiological Record*, **40**, 307.

World Health Organization (1987*a*). *Community health workers: pillars for* *health for all*, Report of the Interregional Conference, Yaoundé, Cameroon, 1–5 December 1986. SHS/CIH/87.2. WHO, Geneva.

World Health Organization (1987*b*). *Community health workers*, Working Document SHS/HMD/SG.87.4. WHO, Geneva.

World Health Organization Study Group (1989). *Strengthening the performance of community health workers in primary health care*, Technical Report Series No. 780. WHO, Geneva.

Wu, Y. M. (1988). Administration of primary health care. In *Chinese health administration*, (ed. R. C. Peng and L. W. Gao), pp. 212–37. Science and Technology Publishing House of Jilin, Changchun. (Chinese).

Wu, Z. and Xiao, J. M. (1988). Bring VHWs' training into standard education system. *Chinese Rural Health Service Administration*, **4**, 12–14.

Xiao, X. W. *et al.* (1988). Carrying out reforms in the township health care system to promote people's health. *Chinese Rural Health Service Administration*, **2**, 32–3.

Zhang, B. Q. (1987). Managerial forms of rural health organisation. *Chinese Rural Health Service Administration*, **11**, 25–8.

Zhang, C. M. (1986). Cooperative medical system under the rural economic reforms. *Chinese Rural Health Service Administration*, **4–5**, 56–9.

Zhou, S. Q. (1984). Barefoot doctors, cooperative medical system. In *Chinese medical encyclopaedia*, pp. 122–124. Shanghai Science and Technology Publishing House, Shanghai.

Zhou, Y. (1986). Experience in the construction of rural health organisations in Yantai City. *Chinese Rural Health Service Administration*, **4–5**, 62–64. (Chinese).

Zhu, A. R. *et al.* (1987). A comparative study of cooperative and privately paid medical systems. In *Health policies and administration*, (ed. Expert Committee on Health Policy and Administration), pp. 51–7. Ministry of Public Health, Beijing.

Zhu, Z. H. (1988). Cooperative medical services. *Chinese Rural Health Service Administration*, **7**, 6–9.

Index